WHEN PREGNANCY AND BIRTH DON'T GO TO PLAN

INSPIRING REAL-LIFE STORIES OF COPING
WITH MISCARRIAGE, INFANT LOSS,
PREMATURE AND SICK NEWBORNS

JO SPICER

BRIGHT
BUTTERFLY

PRAISE FOR THE BOOK "WHEN PREGNANCY AND BIRTH DON'T GO TO PLAN"

INSPIRING REAL-LIFE STORIES OF COPING WITH MISCARRIAGE, INFANT LOSS, PREMATURE AND SICK NEWBORNS

"What a very brave, compassionate and inspiring book. Jo, in this book you have been able to capture the grief, tragedy, joy, love, hope and resilience that the women and their families have experienced.

The stories shared within this book will support health professionals to reflect on how they provide care , what they say and how they respond during such a traumatic and vulnerable time."

— Deborah Cameron, Executive Director of Nursing, Midwifery & Clinical Governance, Illawarra Shoalhaven Local Health District, NSW Health

---

"Jo has again produced a beautifully written account of the experiences that women and their partners face when pregnancy and birth don't unfold as they had hoped and dreamt. Time and time again I was struck by the profound rawness of the grief and suffering the women and their families experienced. The lack of understanding, kindness and compassion from professionals and the broader community often compounded their suffering.

Many of the amazing families in this book managed to develop a strong appreciation of the preciousness of life. Further, many wanted to help and support others and went on to develop creative and beautiful resources and support groups.

This is the human spirit at work; creating value from profound suffering and loss. Thank you Jo and thank you to the women and families for courageously sharing your stories and challenging this taboo subject."

— Dr Sue Leicester, Clinical Psychologist

"Jo has shone the spotlight on many taboo topics that are not always shared and talked about, this is beautiful validation of the experiences many women go through on their journey to be a mother.

Sharing our stories removes the shame hopefully reducing the stigma associated with them and ensuring women can receive the support, empathy, and understanding they deserve."

— Samantha Payne, CEO & Co-Founder, The Pink Elephants Support Network, Miscarriage Support

---

"This collection of very personal and individual stories takes you on a journey that share the experience of loss, of love and of healing.

Jo Spicer has an amazing gift of bringing these invaluable stories to the light sharing something that is most vulnerable and precious. I was walking right alongside these families through each step of their journey. To be allowed into the world of these courageous people was a true honour."

— Dr April Traynor, Family Wellness Chiropractor

CONTENTS

INTRODUCTION

For some of us, having children and creating a family of our own is the single element that gives our lives meaning and purpose. For others of us, having children is optional or perhaps something we don't ever want to do.

No matter how you wish your life to be, the fact remains that women are born with the equipment to one day give birth to babies. We are designed to perform this function and culturally, society has reinforced this biological truth with the ideal that happiness should include perfect offspring. With all the choices available to women today, childless females passing the 30-year mark are still routinely asked by well-meaning friends and family, "When are you going to have kids?"

With opportunities opened up for women in tertiary education in the last 50 years, it was a given that they would use their degrees and diplomas to forge a career rather than immediately looking to exit the workforce to rear children. In Australia, the age of women giving birth to their first child rose from an average of 25 years of age in the 1970s to a high of 31 years of age in 2019.

Delaying pregnancy until later in life can increase the odds of complications, but difficulties with pregnancy and birth can occur at any age. One in four pregnancies results in miscarriage and yet it is still something that is rarely discussed openly. Why? The answer lies somewhere in our cultural history when the role of women was clearly defined as successfully completed by raising children and taking care of the home. If a woman was unable to bear children, her main purpose, did that mean she had failed in life?

Speaking to women from all age ranges, many told me that they had experienced one or more miscarriages but kept it to themselves. They described feelings of failure and inadequacy, thinking that something was wrong with them. It was somehow awful to think that their bodies could not do the most basic task for which it was designed. They blamed themselves for losing their baby even though it had nothing to do with anything they had done.

Some women have difficulties during their pregnancy and give birth to babies who are born struggling to survive and this too creates a minefield of emotional bombshells. Was it something I did? Something I ate? Will my baby die? Could I have done anything differently to prevent this from happening? How did it happen? What went wrong?

I found myself in this position at the birth of my first child. After a very normal pregnancy, I started having contractions one afternoon around three weeks before my due date. Being September, it was peak season for babies and the hospital suggested I stay at home until my contractions were a few minutes apart. The contractions continued all night, but they didn't seem to be increasing or decreasing. By 7am the next morning I had had enough, and we went into hospital.

Upon examination, I was only dilated a few centimetres. This went on until after lunch when my baby's heart rate dropped. I had been in labour for 24 hours. My obstetrician made the call and I was prepped for emergency caesarean* with an epidural*.

It is the most disconcerting sensation—realising that the bottom half of your body is numb and yet totally aware that all of your other senses are fully operational. Even though my body was anaesthetised, I still had the odd feeling of my body being pulled. I could hear my body thumping repeatedly on the operating table as they tried to get my baby out. Her head was wedged in my hip bones and getting her out of that position seemed to me like a tug-o-war!

I remember a nurse whisking my newborn past my face saying, "It's a girl," before taking her away to places unknown. Her father followed her out of theatre, and I was left on the table with the surgeon who was sewing me back together.

Was my baby okay? Questions to the medical staff still in theatre with me were met with uninformative platitudes: "Don't worry, they're taking care of her." Those words did little to calm me. I'd read enough to know that if everything was fine, then right now my baby would be nestled on my chest and we would be having an Instagram moment. That was not what was happening. Instead, my baby was missing in action in some other ward of the hospital while I, her mother, felt powerless, unable to go to her.

They took me to the recovery ward and it was there that I started to shiver. My teeth were chattering so badly that it was impossible to speak. I could not stop shaking no matter how many blankets they put on top of me. Apparently it is one of the side-effects of anaesthetic and though the nurses assured me that it was normal, the fact that they constantly checked my observations made me wonder.

After what seemed like hours, my baby's father came back to recovery to tell me that our newborn was bruised from the extended labour. Her head was too big to fit through my small hips and with every contraction over that 24 hour period, her head was being pushed against my bones. There was no way she would have made it out naturally. When I was finally taken to her, I was shocked to see that her head was literally black and blue from bruising.

We were told that our baby had jaundice*, and that the bruising would make the situation worse because her body would have the added burden of breaking down the haemoglobin as part of the healing process. The haemoglobin is broken down into bilirubin* which is then processed by the liver and with the extreme bruising, our little girl would need help so as not to reach a life-threatening level of bilirubin.

The treatment was phototherapy* requiring our newborn to be placed under special blue light. This was back in the days before humidicribs, so she lay in something that looked like an open planter box with lights shining on her.

There was nothing we could do but sit beside her little box, hoping and praying that she would improve. Her bilirubin levels kept climbing despite the light therapy, and the paediatrician talked to us about the possibility of requiring a total blood exchange transfusion where 100% of our baby's blood would be removed and replaced by someone else's blood.

It just so happened that I had a friend who had required this procedure as a newborn. Now in her 30s she shared that she had been sick with different ailments her entire life and she attributed it all to the blood exchange transfusion. She advised us to do anything we could to prevent this from happening to our baby.

This information added more stress to our watch and wait. For two weeks we sat there, powerless to do anything but hope for improvement. I would have swapped places with her in a heartbeat.

We reached the point where the doctor told us the blood exchange transfer was a necessity. We asked for a little more time and thankfully, a few hours later her levels began to drop just a little. Slowly but surely, they continued to fall and eventually they reached a place where the hospital staff were happy for us to take her home. Today she is a happy and healthy 24-year-old enjoying life to the fullest, travelling and working overseas.

Five years later, I fell pregnant with my second child. At 14 weeks, I caught a virus that seemed to be going around our circle of family and friends. Most people seemed to cough and suffer the usual cold and flu symptoms and then recover after a couple of weeks. I was the exception, and after two weeks I was only getting worse. My cough persisted and became so intense that I was having severe pain in my ribs area every time I coughed. I lost my voice and eventually was hospitalised.

A respiratory specialist diagnosed that I had effectively shredded my lungs and bruised my ribs with the excessive coughing and that was the cause of all the pain. I had a serious illness but treating me caused a dilemma—the medications doctors normally would prescribe could harm my baby. But if I didn't get well, how would I nourish my baby? It was a real chicken vs egg problem.

Over the course of my pregnancy, I was given some nine different medications in an attempt to heal me while keeping my baby healthy. They were largely ineffective, and I was sick for most of the pregnancy.

At 35 weeks' gestation, I talked to my obstetrician about my first pregnancy. She was a different obstetrician than my first one, and I explained that it was likely that this baby's head would be too big for a vaginal birth and that we probably needed a planned caesarean.

Based on this information she sent me for an ultrasound and we were all stunned when we viewed the measurements—my baby already had the average head size of a 42 week old baby at 35 weeks!

There was no question this baby needed to come out and we went in for an elective caesarean the following week. Everything proceeded well, the obstetrician cutting along the same scar line from my first birth. My baby boy was delivered and put straight into a humidicrib as he also had jaundice. He responded well and did not escalate to the levels of his sister. It was discovered that he had an ABO Incompatibility* that contributed to his jaundice but fortunately, it was not severe.

We were worried about the effect of my health issues and the medication I took during pregnancy. He was immediately placed under the care of a paediatrician and soon after birth was diagnosed with severe asthma.*

For the first six months of his life, we barely slept, keeping one ear open for any signs of breathing difficulties. There were countless times that we drove to Westmead Children's Hospital in the middle of the night when our home asthma protocol was no longer effective and we required urgent specialist care.

When you know the emergency triage nurses by name and are immediately ushered through to the inner sanctum without sitting for hours in the waiting room with everyone else, you know that the situation is serious. We were routinely fast tracked through so that our baby could be hooked up to oxygen and administered steroids to get his lungs working.

I remember one night when we rushed to hospital, asking my parents to look after our five-year-old daughter overnight. As expected, we were admitted and transferred to the ward. The next morning, my son's dad stayed with him while I went home to get some fresh clothes. I arrived home and noticed an itch all around my torso. I had a look and it was a huge rash. I had shingles.

Because shingles is the same disease as chickenpox, I was not allowed back into the hospital. My doctor advised me to leave my daughter with my parents, and so I was home alone with an excruciating case of shingles that felt something like being stabbed with a sharp knife while being so itchy I wanted to scratch off my skin but I couldn't because it hurt too much to touch.

It was one of my lowest moments. My immune system was shot as a result of the strain of the pregnancy and then the sleepless nights caring for my newborn son. I was frustrated because I was the one supposed to be caring for my children and I was incapacitated and unable to do my job.

Eventually I healed and my son came out of hospital. The paediatrician explained that our baby's lungs could not cope with the changes in temperature in Sydney and asked if we could move to a more temperate climate. As we both worked for ourselves, the option was a real possibility and within six months we moved 1000km north to Queensland.

The move proved positive for my son's health. We added chiropractic care and naturopathy to his treatment and within a couple of years he was much improved, using medication only on an occasional basis. Today he is a thriving and healthy 19-year-old planning on an engineering career.

As much as we all wish pregnancy and birth would go perfectly to plan, just like the rest of life it doesn't always turn out that way. How do we deal with the curve balls that come our way? What is the best way to cope when we are faced with indescribable tragedy and loss?

There are no right or wrong ways to deal with these traumatic events in our lives. Whatever you feel is real and valid. I am not here to tell you what to do or how to be. What I hope I can do for you is to present the stories of women who have bravely faced a huge range of issues around pregnancy and birth. Read their stories and find out what they have done to deal with their trauma in their own way. You may not relate to all of the stories but some of them might resonate strongly with you and give you the strength and courage to cope a little better with your own situation.

I want to thank each and every one of the brave families who have shared their stories in these pages. They are all from Australia as am I, so I have used Australian spelling and language. Throughout the book you will find particular medical references marked with an asterisk upon their first mention. I have included a simple terminology index as an appendix to explain their meaning.

If you have been challenged in falling pregnant or carrying a baby to term; if you have suffered miscarriage or loss; if you have struggled with a difficult birth, premature babies or sick babies; or if you are dealing with post-natal depression or anxiety, know that you are not alone and that there are people and organisations available to support you.

My greatest hope is that this book will give you the strength to survive, the inspiration to revive and the will to move forward with your life and thrive.

Jo Spicer

1

TAHYNA

- Three miscarriages
- Gestational Diabetes*
- Rainbow baby* Echo, aged four
- Rainbow baby Oisin, aged one
- Postnatal Anxiety*

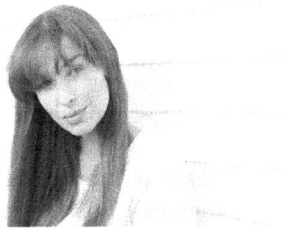

Award winning director, writer and actress—none of these roles prepared Tahyna for the intense sadness and overwhelming joy of motherhood.

A veteran of the entertainment industry, Tahyna began modelling when she was just eight years old. By her late teens, she was a regular on our screens as Perri Lowe in the Australian TV series, Blue Water High and major films including X-Men Origins.

It was a natural progression for Tahyna to move behind the camera, writing and directing films inspired by her personal experiences.

> **"A part of me was frustrated that I had no more control as an actress. I love it (acting), but nothing fulfils me more than when I put all the pieces together behind the scenes."**

In 2014, Tahyna wrote and directed a semi-autobiographical film called Oren. This short film received official selection in both US and European film festivals, winning Best International Short Film at the prestigious Hollywood Reel Independent Film Festival.

"I wish I'd said something. I wish I had told the sonographer, 'Don't call it, it.' I just wish I'd said something, so she realised the impact of her words."

Later that night, the couple sat through an awkward dinner with their roommates who did not know about the pregnancy. It was obvious that Tahyna had been crying but they all tried to act normally.

Then one of them asked jokingly, "So are you pregnant yet?" Tahyna remembers tears filling her eyes as she forced a laugh and retreated to her bedroom, leaving Tristan to explain that they had just lost the baby.

The couple had no idea how to process the loss. Tahyna was still hopeful the next day, taking another pregnancy test and saying to Tristan, "It's still positive!" But then she started searching the internet and realised that the baby was gone and that the test was only registering the pregnancy hormone still in her body.

"I didn't lose pregnancy matter, or whatever, I lost a baby. I had already planned everything in my head. The next 50 years had flown through my brain."

Tahyna's family wanted to support her, but they were not sure what she needed.

"My family, bless them, just didn't know what to say and do. No one thought it would happen to me, and no one would talk about it anyway. Mum said to me, 'I had a miscarriage it's pretty common,' and that type of thing. She was trying to come up with solutions, but she wasn't equipped to deal with how I was going to handle it."

From speaking to other women who have experienced miscarriage, Tahyna understands that words such as those expressed by her mother, have cut other women deeply. This was not the case for Tahyna—she did not feel that they were dismissive of her pain, but rather that they were reassuring her that this was not the end.

Looking back, Tahyna now recognises that nothing could have helped her at that point. She did, however, greatly appreciate that her sister, Cheyenne, flew over to spend time with her. Cheyenne did the only thing that she could, and that was to physically be there for support.

One of the most emotionally difficult things Tahyna had to do was to tell Tristan's parents.

"I remember I felt humiliated to tell Tristan's parents, because I've always tried so hard to be the perfect daughter-in-law. That really hurt. I really did not want to tell them that I failed. That was really tough to swallow."

Tahyna decided to take some time off, joining Tristan on a work stint in Ireland. She spent that time struggling with her waves of emotions, trying to heal and come to terms with her trauma.

"I was so sad. I was so, so sad. I blamed myself, I thought something was wrong, or I'd done something wrong. We hadn't tried again, so I thought, 'Is this going to be a thing with me now? Does this mean that this is going to be my path now?' I was so upset. I just really wanted a baby, but I had so much fear."

Shortly after returning from Ireland, Tristan and Tahyna moved to London. To increase their chances of a successful pregnancy, they made health a priority. Tristan quit drinking and they both started a regime of supplements. Little did they know that they were already pregnant—somewhere in the moving process, they had spontaneously conceived!

Tahyna armed herself with knowledge, researching everything she could find out about pregnancy and birth.

"That pregnancy, especially early on, was very, very scary. I had an early ultrasound at six weeks, and by that stage, I was like a pro, I knew everything about ultrasounds, blood tests and what I needed, so I was kind of telling the doctor, I drove the doctor nuts."

Everything was right on track. Tahyna's blood tests showed her HCG levels* had doubled and the ultrasound showed her 'tiny blob.'

"I remember turning to Tristan with my little blob on my piece of paper and saying, 'She looks like she's wearing sunglasses.' And I knew she was a girl. I was already, straight away, emotionally attached like you wouldn't believe."

Even though every indication showed that her pregnancy was progressing beautifully, Tahyna admits that she went a 'little loopy'. She became obsessive with ultrasounds, having another at nine weeks, then again at 12 weeks. Her General Practitioner (GP)* in London encouraged her to relax and enjoy the pregnancy, but this was difficult for Tahyna to do. Her miscarriage had created a fear in her that she could not shake.

A film project in Australia bought Tahyna back home. Her morning sickness was out of control, but after the 20 weeks scan, when she could see her baby clearly, she had a period where she did not panic and felt genuinely elated.

At 30 week's gestation, the baby's measurements showed that she had stopped growing. Tahyna was rushed to the hospital and given steroids. Her doctor urged her to consider delivery via caesarean section, but Tahyna felt so in tune with the pregnancy with a strong sense that everything was going to be fine, so she asked the doctors to give it a few days before making a decision.

Sure enough, the steroids worked well, and the baby had a big growth spurt. Baby stayed in place and finally, after a natural labour, Echo arrived in the world.

> **"Echo was a totally healthy baby, she was a normal baby, bad sleeper, the usual, but a perfectly healthy and relaxed baby. I was like, I could have 10 of you."**

Tahyna and Tristan continued their careers while raising Echo. Around 18 months later, just after Tahyna finished work on a short film, the family travelled to Ireland. Both Tristan and Tahyna felt strong and healthy, and decided it was a good time to try for another child.

She is not sure how, but Tahyna has always been able to tell when she is ovulating. Again, they fell pregnant straight away and this was verified by the morning sickness! Tahyna felt confident about the pregnancy, taking a photo of Echo holding a positive test. Two days before Christmas 2017, they had their first ultrasound and could not find a heartbeat, but the sonographer suggested that perhaps their dates were wrong, so they didn't worry.

It was so exciting to share their news with family and friends over the Christmas break. Their next scan was scheduled for 12 weeks and it was heart-wrenching to discover that there was a foetus but no heartbeat.

> **"That totally broke me. I remember sitting in there, trying to be very pragmatic about it. My initial thing is to always be, OK, give me all of the information and I'll just deal with this. I've always sort of been like that with everything. But when the technician left the room, I was just sobbing with Tristan**

because again, I had imagined everything. I had made this thing in my head and it wasn't meant to be."

This experience became the trigger for Tahyna's next film: M.O.M. Misunderstandings of Miscarriage. She had so many emotions running through her and wanted to talk about them but wasn't sure if she was ready to hear anyone else's opinion. So, she decided to express her raw feelings to the camera, in the form of a video diary.

"I really had no idea why I was doing it. But when Tristan asked, 'Do you want to go anywhere?' I said, 'I want to lock myself in a room, because I'm too scared to tell anyone that this has happened again, and I don't want to deal with it.' I felt so conflicted about everything, so I started filming."

Tahyna's doctor advised her to let the pregnancy pass naturally. She went home and waited, and waited, and waited. A week passed and nothing happened. She had another blood test and discovered that her HCG levels were still rising. Her morning sickness was still intense, and in every way, Tahyna's body continued to experience all the signs of pregnancy.

Tahyna was baffled—what her mind knew to be true was different to what her body was doing. These symptoms continued for three weeks until she was out at lunch, and she started to bleed.

The bleeding was heavy and continuous. With no information or forewarning of what to expect, Tahyna accepted the process as normal. After five week of blood loss, her iron levels and the volume of blood in her body was so low, she was almost anaemic*. Realising that she was very sick, Tahyna went to her GP and he referred her to a private obstetrician.

The couple was informed that the pregnancy had not been expelled properly. The doctor showed them pictures and it was traumatising to see the shape of their baby. He was kind enough to acknowledge the loss before recommending a dilation and curettage (D & C)* procedure.

"It was horrible, it was just an awful, it felt invasive. I remember going into the hospital and the anaesthetist said, 'I'm just going to need your credit card details, I'll put you to sleep, and then your doctor will come in and then you'll be out in three hours, and then you can have dinner.' It felt like I was being processed."

Tahyna continued recording her journey, asking Tristan to film her in hospital, immediately after the D & C.

"For him, it was a bit like, I don't know why you're doing this, but for me, I wasn't sure what I was going to do with all of this stuff, but I knew I had to do something with it."

The filming process helped Tahyna to focus her thoughts on what she was actually feeling emotionally. She realised that she was not dealing with the grief, self-blame, guilt and shame. She didn't feel that she could talk about her miscarriage, and in the midst of her own trauma, she began to wonder how many other women were feeling the same way.

"That thought was a trigger for me, recognising that maybe I have to do this for the greater good, for someone else, so that they don't have to feel what I'm feeling."

Tahyna began talking to other women. She embarked on a journey to discover why the shame, stigma and taboo exists around the subject of miscarriage. It was important for her to get right down to the 'nitty gritty' of how this thinking developed and why it continues.

"It's an individual process, but I think deep down, it's ingrained in women that it is our job to bear children. I think it goes way back to past generations as well. This is a secret women's business type of thing, where we deal with it all on our own, and we try and carry on as best as we can."

Even though each person Tahyna met had dealt with miscarriage in their own way, she learnt that even in today's society, where women have every opportunity choose their own path, that a woman's identity is still tied to her ability to bear children.

"What I've noticed is that self-blame and guilt is really strong. Many women believe that, 'My role as a woman is to have children and if I can't, then what am I?' And the other thing is the longing to be a mother. If there is no proof of a child, then does that make you not a mother?"

Opening up the conversation about miscarriage and pregnancy loss is a driving force for Tahyna. She truly believes that if she can shift the thinking about this issue and bring it out from behind closed doors, then her personal journey has happened for a reason.

"I feel like I specifically went through miscarriages to make this film. It was great when we saw a perinatal* psychologist, because she said, 'Often mothers who were very attached to

their child or their foetus find great healing in honouring that child, whether planting a flower, or getting a little bracelet or something for that child.' And this film is for the babies that I lost. That's how I look at it."

Tahyna found that the key commonalities amongst many women were feelings of isolation, a lack of information provided by the medical system and a lack of information in wider society, with friends and families not knowing how to provide support.

"I hope that women are given resources and effective tools to deal with what they are going through, both physically and emotionally. I also really, really hope that generations to come don't feel like it's a burden that they have to carry alone, and that they feel ashamed to talk about. I just really hope that we become more open about pregnancy loss."

While working on the documentary, Tahyna and Tristan tried again to conceive. They fell pregnant in June 2018 but within days of discovering she was pregnant, Tahyna started bleeding. She woke up pregnant and went to bed no longer pregnant—it was another loss.

"It was the lowest of lows. I was on set working, I was directing, so there was no way I could be like, 'Oh guys, I need to leave.' I had to stay there until the very end, and it was just, I remember just feeling like I was in a marshmallow world. What I mean by that is everything was fluffy and fuzzy. I just couldn't really grasp anything that day."

For a while, Tahyna could not even think about falling pregnant. She felt completely unprepared to go through it again. Tristan was just as affected by the miscarriages, but as a man, he handled things differently.

"We shed many tears together at those ultrasounds, but he's always felt, 'I have to be a rock.' It's in his DNA. It's not something men want to sit around a bar and talk about. They also need our strength and support as well. This is where the whole conversation needs to be opened up, because we need to work together, like anything, as a human race, it's not just a women's issue, it's a human issue, it's a social human issue."

For the weeks following their third miscarriage, Tristan and Tahyna did not try to conceive, nor did they prevent conception. Two months later, they discovered they were pregnant again.

Tahyna's pregnancy developed throughout filming of the documentary and she recalled how difficult it was to meet and film women about pregnancy loss while her own tummy got bigger.

> **"It was so hard because I knew how lucky I was, but I also wanted to tell them how terrified I was, but I didn't want to tell them, it was so conflicting... I remember Tristan being worried about me because I would come home in tears, because I'd spoke to a woman who lost her baby at 35 weeks, and he said, 'Why are you doing this? Maybe don't do this right now.' But I knew I had to keep going."**

The pregnancy progressed well, though Tahyna did suffer gestational diabetes*. Toward the end of the pregnancy, an ultrasound showed that the baby could have Hydrocephalus*, an abnormal enlargement of the brain cavities, also known as ventricles. Tahyna started researching and found some terrifying results including severe disability and death. They had to wait two weeks for another scan, riding on a rollercoaster of emotions. The new scan showed no change. There was nothing else they could do except wait until the baby was born.

Thankfully, the baby was healthy and with great joy, they welcomed Oisin to the family in March 2019. Nonetheless, after the anxieties of the pregnancy, Tahyna was worried about his well-being.

> **"I was micro-managing. I think I had a form of post-natal anxiety or depression because I was micro-managing every little movement, his eye contact, everything. I was putting so much pressure on me and him because of the fear."**

Oisin had been suffering with colic*, but the day we met he was blissfully sleeping in his mother's arms after breastfeeding. Tahyna suspected he had allergies to certain foods, and she was eliminating food groups from her diet to prevent their transmission to him through her breast milk. Every day he improved and at three months, Oisin looked the picture of health.

Tahyna recognises how blessed she is to have her incredible husband and beautiful family. Echo and Oisin are everything to her and she loves being a mum, so much so that they are contemplating adding another child, perhaps not through pregnancy, but adoption.

Life is all about balance for Tahyna as she juggles parenting and her passion to make meaningful documentaries and creative film projects. There is absolutely no doubt that she is doing it brilliantly.

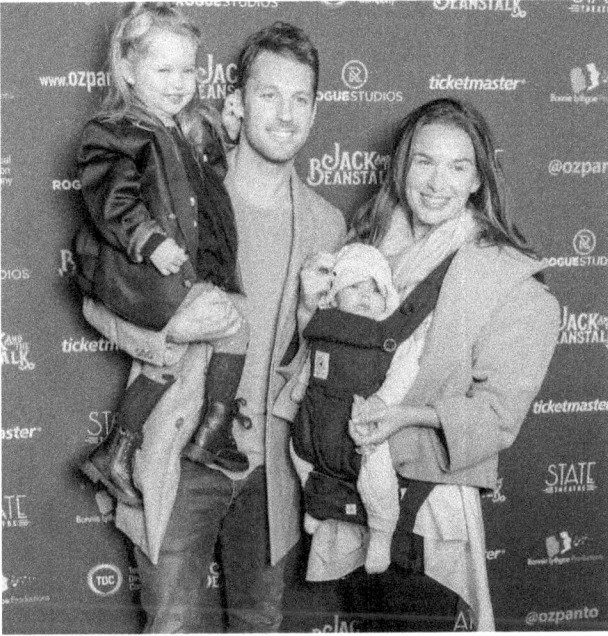

Tahyna, Tristan, Echo and Oisin

"Really be aware of where that person's sitting. Really, really take the time to listen to them, before you react or try and come up with a solution, because that will clue you in on who they are and what they need. Respect their grief, respect their process, and respect what they have been through, their trauma."

2

KATE AND CRYSTAL

- Cervical Cancer
- In Vitro Fertilisation (IVF)*
- Sperm Donor
- Egg Transfer
- Early Medical Menopause
- Lymphoedema*

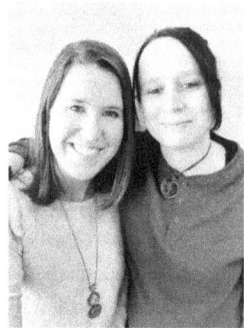

Kate has truly found her calling in the NSW Police Force. As a detective, she has exceptional investigative skills, but it is her infectious smile, kindness and genuine caring nature that immediately puts you at ease. These attributes come from her grounded upbringing as part of a tight-knit family in the Illawarra, a regional area south of Sydney.

Training for her chosen career started with several years at the New South Wales Police Academy in the country town of Goulburn.

> **"I loved it because there was a group of eight or nine of us girls who all lived together in town. It was a full college experience except that there were many more rope runs, sit-ups and push-ups!"**

Amongst the group was fellow trainee, Crystal. The two became friends, graduated and then went their separate ways—Crystal to a coastal town called Coffs Harbour, and Kate to the city suburb of Maroubra.

Located in the Eastern Suburbs of Sydney, Maroubra Police Station was a busy workplace. Kate was thrown in the deep end, learning on the job and acclimatising to a fast-paced lifestyle. Her superior officers noticed her initiative and diligence in investigations and encouraged her to aim higher. Kate successfully completed the Detective's Course and became designated in 2017.

The job was non-stop and involved dealing with a variety of very different situations. Some of them took an emotional toll, but Kate was able to compartmentalise these events to keep going. In 2017, she investigated a number of particularly gruelling cases including one that was absolutely horrific.

A young couple was driving south as part of a convoy of cars with their friends. They took a corner too quickly, causing the car to flip and explode into flames. The couple could not get out of the car and even though their friends pulled over to help, the fire prevented them from saving their lives.

> **"One of the uniform cars was first on the scene. Hearing him on the radio, screaming for help with their friends all there…it was horrendous. They both died, burned alive in the car. We cordoned off the road as a crime scene, and shortly after, the parents of the couple arrived while the car was still on fire. I had to deliver the death messages to these two families. Normally, when you deliver a death message to a family you are 100% certain that the person has died. I had to do it while they were watching their loved ones burn in the car."**

The communication was complicated by language barriers. The girl's mother was Macedonian, the boy's father was Lebanese, and neither were completely fluent in English. At one point, the boy's father broke through crime scene barrier and ran towards his son, burning in the car.

> **"We were at the scene for 10 hours and it was heartbreaking. Absolutely heartbreaking. We don't usually follow up with families, but on this occasion, all the officers that were there went to the funeral. Afterwards, I just shut down and even now, the smell of chemical fire still affects me."**

For Kate, it was the straw that broke the camel's back. She needed a creative outlet, to do something completely removed from her work.

> **"I love my job and I think that I'm good at my job. I think I'm good for the community, the families and the people I work for and with. But I needed a break. So I went to a beading**

workshop around the corner from me. For those two hours a week that I was there, I wasn't a cop."

The other thing that Kate did was to reach out to her friend Crystal. Between shift work and living at opposite ends of the state, the two had only seen each other a handful of times since training at the Academy, but one day, out of the blue, Kate felt the urge to reach out. The two girls arranged to reconnect and from that moment on, they realised that they felt more than friendship.

"We have so much respect for one another and each other's histories. We already knew each other as friends when we got together. It was kind of one thing after another and all of a sudden when it happened, it was it. She's such a beautiful, beautiful human."

In 2017, Crystal proposed, just prior to the Australian Marriage Law Postal Survey designed to gauge support for legalising same-sex marriage. The plebiscite stirred strong beliefs that were voiced through media, social media, politicians and groups on both sides of the issue. The couple thought that the legislation would never pass and decided to go ahead and book a venue for the following February. If necessary, they would have a commitment ceremony instead of a wedding.

To their surprise, the plebiscite returned a 61.6% 'Yes' response and the government legislation legalising same-sex marriage came into effect on 9 December. When the couple heard the news, Crystal was overwhelmed.

"She looked at me and it was as if her life flashed before her eyes. I reminded her that she was the one who proposed to me. She was freaking out, saying, "Oh my god, this is real! We're actually getting legally married!""

Kate and Crystal were one of the first couples to be married under the new legislation. The day was a perfect celebration of family and friends, with the mum of one of Kate's friends, a civil celebrant, conducting the ceremony. Kate feels that one of the best parts of their decision is being able to call each other 'wife'.

"It gives us a sense of normalcy that everyone can relate to. We are just like every other married couple. It's the simplicity of being able to explain my relationship by saying, 'This is my wife.' It's not, I'm gay or I'm same sex or whatever. It says,

'This is the person that I love and I've chosen to spend the rest of my life with her.' That's all that matters."

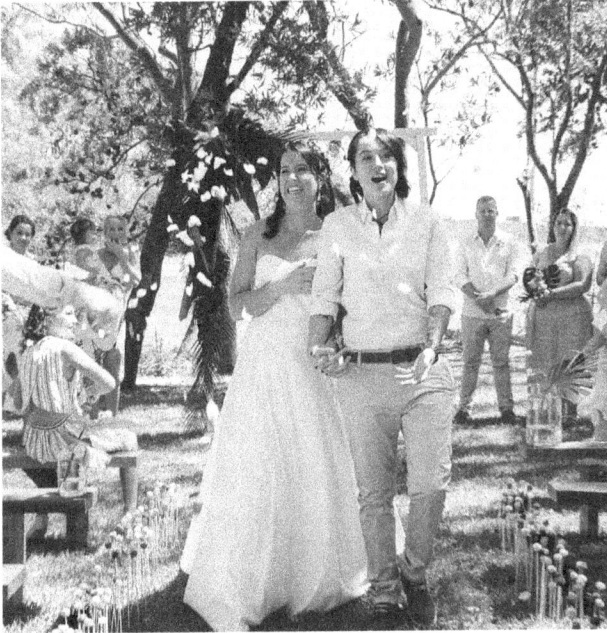

Kate and Crystal's wedding

As soon as they married, Crystal was ready to start a family. They had decided to use IVF and knowing it would be expensive, Kate thought it would be good to keep working for a while to save up for the procedure. She also wanted to do some travel before settling down, so they agreed to wait a year.

It was a busy 12 months with big life changes, including a relocation to Garah, a tiny town in country NSW with a population of 300 people. The nearest town centre is Moree, located an hour's drive away.

Crystal and Kate were warmly welcomed into the friendly community, with locals pleased to get a "two-for-one" deal of two police officers for the price of one transfer. For Kate, it was a huge change from living in the bustling city of Sydney.

Up to that point in her life, Kate was a healthy, active woman who had never required medical care. She told me how ironic it was that when medical care was easily accessible, she didn't need it but as soon as she moved to the middle of nowhere, it became essential.

Kate started to notice a constant pain on the left-hand side of her groin. It didn't seem like a strained muscle and it didn't improve, so she went to the doctor to have it checked. After some tests and an examination, she was diagnosed with gluten intolerance.

"I didn't eat gluten for six months. The doctor had an attitude that it was just one of those things that women have and that it was just my lot in life."

Apart from her dietary change, Kate didn't think much of it until they decided to start IVF around the time of their first wedding anniversary. The nearest clinic was in Brisbane, a five-hour drive away from their new home.

Their initial consultation with the doctor involved preparation for the procedure, including the question of who would carry the baby. It was always going to be Kate.

"I had romanticised pregnancy. All I wanted to do was get big, have big boobs and float around my pool and feel the baby. I wasn't that certain on motherhood, but I was really certain that I wanted to get pregnant."

This was the perfect fit for Crystal. Even though she was excited to become a mother, carrying a baby had never figured into her life plan. Kate explained that for Crystal, her body is a sacred space and that the changes that pregnancy brings are not ones that she wanted to experience.

As part of the checks and tests prior to starting IVF, the doctor asked if either of them had recently had a pap smear. Both of them were overdue for the test by about 12 months so the doctor offered to do it for both of them while they were there.

As she was examining Kate, the doctor was not happy with what she saw. She referred her to a specialist for a biopsy* done before the couple made the long drive home. A few days later while she was at work, the doctor's secretary called Kate to say that the doctor needed to go through the results. She advised Kate to go home so the couple could be together for the discussion. Kate works 50km from home and that phone call was like a warning to brace for bad news.

She raced home and the couple sat in front of the screen, talking to the doctor via Skype.

"This poor IVF doctor who is obviously not normally delivering this type of diagnosis to people, says, 'You've got cervical

cancer.' And I said, 'OK, that's cool, what are we doing? What's the plan, the next step? Is this going to push back the IVF timeline?'"

Kate took the news calmly because around that time, quite a few of her friends had received abnormal pap smear results, diagnoses of polyps and some had even required LLETZ* surgery. She thought that it would be a simple and quick procedure, a little bump in the road before they started on the serious task of conceiving a baby. But the doctor's face was ashen as she explained the seriousness of the situation.

"She said, 'Kate, this isn't about whether or not you can have a baby. This is about whether or not you survive.' And that was it. I just lost it."

For Kate the following five days felt like a blur. She had just been given a life-threatening diagnosis and was being told that she needed to find an oncologist. She didn't even know what an oncologist was and there certainly wasn't one available in Garah.

"It was the bleakest time because I didn't have any answers. If you've got a plan, if you've got something to work towards, it's manageable. You can work that in your head. But if you've got nothing and no one is talking to you because they don't know the answers, that's the worst. And that's what I tell people who reach out to me—just get through those first few days of nothingness."

Kate is a self-confessed "Type A Personality"—highly organised, competitive, ambitious, impatient and highly aware of time management. She had applied all of these traits to planning her life with a checklist of things that needed to be done for her to be happy. Now all of that was under threat.

"I thought I needed to tick the boxes—have the kids, the wife, the money, the house and then I'd be happy and enjoying myself. But something like this makes you go, well, I might not get all of that. Nothing is guaranteed. I remember just sobbing to my wife, just crying and saying over and over, 'I don't want to die.'"

The nearest oncologist was located in Brisbane, almost 500m from home. Kate is grateful that her mum, a nurse by profession, flew up to accompany them to their appointment with the cancer specialist. She was an enormous help to both Kate and Crystal, taking on the role of primary support person.

> **"Mum was obviously stressed as well, but for Crystal, I imagine just how difficult it is when you've got a partner going through a cancer diagnosis. You can't always rely on them to be taking everything in and to understand because they're scared as well."**

The first step was to undergo an Examination Under Anaesthetic (EUA)*. After the doctor performed the exploratory procedure, she informed Kate and her family that the cancer appeared to be confined to the cervix. Her recommendation was a trachelectomy*, the surgical removal of the cervix rather than a hysterectomy so that potentially, in the future, she would be able to carry a baby. If they got to that stage, then Kate would likely require cervical cerclage*, procedures used to suture the lower part of the uterus shut to maintain the pregnancy.

> **"That's how fixed I was on carrying a baby, that I was willing to do that as opposed to a full hysterectomy*, getting it out and just getting on with my life."**

Kate started searching the internet for any information on a trachelectomy. She could barely find anything, so she continued her quest on social media and typed "#trachelectomy" on Instagram. This action connected her with a Brisbane woman of similar age who had already undergone the procedure. The two women bonded over their shared experience and their friendship continues today.

> **"We talk all the time. Through her I was able to find out about the procedure. Not just what was going to happen on the operating table, but everything afterwards."**

Her PET scan* supported the doctor's opinion that the cancer was fully contained in the cervix. To be sure, the doctor advised that they would also remove the associated lymph nodes just in case. This gave Kate the confidence to go into surgery trusting that the cancer would be removed from her body and that she would soon be back on track with her life plan.

Kate's operation went well. It required a large incision from hip to hip and she needed a few days in hospital before going home to recover. In the meantime, her oncologist sent her tissue samples for testing. Eight lymph nodes were clear and one that had a six-millimetre cancerous deposit.

The treatment for this condition is intense chemotherapy and radiation. For anyone facing this regime the prospect is daunting, but for Kate it was devastating—it would forever destroy her ability to carry a baby.

As the couple tried to grapple with what they were being told, the oncologist outlined an action plan that would give them some hope. She was aware that Kate had been referred from an IVF doctor and understood how much they wanted a child.

> **"My amazing oncologist said to me, 'It will make you infertile, so I will give you one round of IVF before the radiation and chemo. Now that we know it's in your lymph nodes, I don't want to leave it too long before we start. Whatever eggs you get or you don't get, that's it.'"**

This tiny window of time was Kate's only chance to ever be able to have a biological child. The couple didn't have time to think about it, they just had to go ahead and put things in motion.

It was not a good starting point for IVF. Before even thinking about the hormone injections required in preparation for egg harvesting, a woman usually does everything she can to be in peak physical health. Kate's body was in the worst state of her life—she had the anaesthetic from two recent surgeries in her system plus all the drugs that were administered as part of those operations. She was still recovering from the surgery and emotionally dealing with her upcoming cancer treatment and the side-effects. Her body was in no shape to create optimal numbers of good quality eggs.

> **"We were both getting so overwhelmed. I said to Crystal, 'We can only do one step at a time. Let's not look too far ahead. Let's just get the eggs out and put them on ice.' Otherwise, you look ahead and start thinking, 'I need to organise my will and my funeral and all sorts of stuff.'"**

By not getting caught up in what could have been or what will be, the couple focused on what they needed to do in the present. As soon as she was sufficiently recovered, Kate started the IVF hormone injections into her stomach which was difficult and painful for her to do. When they were told to come in for harvesting, Kate worried about the condition of her eggs and, knowing that only about 35% of those would become embryos, she was also anxious about the number they would retrieve.

The procedure yielded five eggs that had to be fertilised immediately. In the rush to get the cycle done, Kate and Crystal had not previously chosen a sperm donor and they were told they had to pick one straight away.

"The sperm was a big deal to us. We thought we would get a book with heaps of donors and photos and we could take our time and choose one. But in the end, we had about 15 to choose from and all they had was a little bio, highest level of education, why they wanted to be a sperm donor, and a little bit about their medical history. We ended up picking one who had no cancer in his immediately family. We might as well have drawn them out of a hat."

The five eggs were fertilised and then came the wait to find out how many would survive.

"They called me every day from the lab to say, 'Another one's died.' Another one's died. By the end of the five days, there was only one little egg."

Each day, with each phone call, it felt like a little more of her dream died with the embryo. On top of the toll this took on her emotionally, Kate was simultaneously being marked up for radiotherapy. The oncologist insisted that they move quickly and, as is standard, patients are marked with permanent tattoos to assist the therapists to aim the radiation precisely.

"My radiation mark-up was a really traumatic tattooing. I've got quite a few tattoos, but to have that done was a really, really surprisingly traumatic experience. I've always found tattoos to be empowering. They are my choice to have on my body, even if it's something that you later regret or if you fall out of love with them. It was a decision you made at the time to have some control over your body. Having yourself permanently tattooed, to line you up under a machine that's basically going to deviate your life from the path you had set for yourself, that you can never not have on your body, it affected me more than I thought."

Their precious embryo was put on ice while Kate underwent her treatment. Due to the fact that daily clinic visits were required, she needed to temporarily move to a major town. There is an excellent cancer centre near Kate's childhood home so they chose be treated there where they could stay with family.

Treatment involved 28 days of radiation and five rounds of weekly chemotherapy. The radiation began well, but the longer it went on, the worse the side-effects became.

"It's like sunburn on steroids. It was pelvic radiation so after a while, my skin disintegrated. I couldn't sit down. I couldn't wear underwear. I felt like crap from the chemo and this was happening as well. I still had to do things like go to the bathroom and it was horrendous. My skin was just falling off, like I was rotting from the inside."

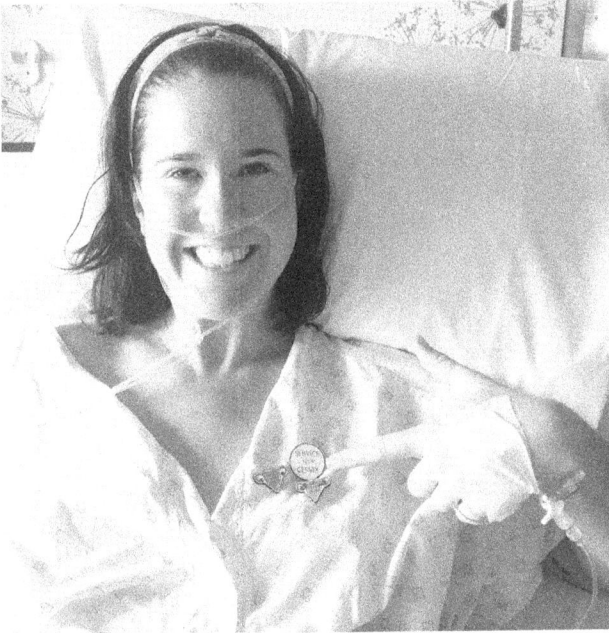

Kate during cancer treatment

The treatment took a huge toll on her body but Crystal was there to support Kate through every moment. It took months for her to heal internally from the surgery, and even longer for her skin to repair.

Radiation has rendered Kate's reproductive organs inoperable. She no longer has her period and is dealing with menopause and all of its symptoms at the age of 32. She has heat waves that feel like bands of fire across her lower back that move upward and out of the top of her head. Her doctor has prescribed a gel hormone treatment and Kate combines this with acupuncture sessions to ease the hot flushes.

These symptoms only serve to underline the fact that, despite her hopes and dreams and the plans she had made with Crystal, she will never experience pregnancy.

"On top of everything I was going through, I was also mourning not being able to carry a pregnancy. Because for me, it was a really important part of my identity. On Instagram there's these beautiful glowing women with their bump photos. I started seeing a psychologist who is amazing and has really helped me."

Kate fully believes in the benefits of being able to talk about your trauma. She personally finds it therapeutic in maintaining her mental health and she encourages others to do the same with a professional or trusted friend.

Both women knew that the obvious solution for their embryo was for Crystal to carry the baby, but knowing how she felt about it, Kate made a point of never putting pressure on her to do it. She recalled their initial appointment to start IVF when the doctor asked Crystal if she would carry the baby if anything happened to Kate.

"We laughed. We were like, 'Oh god, what kind of alternate universe would we be living in?' We were so smug."

It turned out that Crystal didn't need any prompting. She came to the realisation herself and offered, saying to Kate, "Let's just try it and see if it happens. Then if it happens, we'll do everything else."

In November 2019, two months after Kate's cancer treatment ended, Crystal had their embryo implanted. They were told not to do any home pregnancy tests and to wait for two weeks to do a blood test. The couple couldn't wait that long, so Crystal brought some pregnancy tests home. They did six tests and they were all positive.

Feeling confident, they went for the blood test and received a call with the results. The lab technician told them that Crystal was not pregnant.

"And literally, Crystal had one hand on the Bundy rum! I said, 'We've just done six pregnancy tests and I'm pretty sure she's pregnant.' The lab tech went off to double-check the results and came back on the phone. 'Sorry, it was the wrong test. You are actually pregnant.' She told me the hCG levels and I got off the phone and started Googling—the levels were in the twin to triplet range. I didn't tell Crystal because I was thinking, 'Oh my god, she didn't want to get pregnant in the first place. If she's pregnant with twins or triplets she's going to kill me!'"

Kate couldn't help but think that before she had been so worried about not getting a baby at all, and now she was worried about having too many! She managed to keep the information to herself until their first dating scan where the sonographer confirmed there was just one baby.

The couple is not surprised that their embryo implanted—Crystal comes from a family of very fertile women and is one of five daughters. All of the scans to date have shown a perfectly healthy baby, growing beautifully. But for Crystal and Kate, it is not the pregnancy they envisaged.

> **"This is the interesting thing that we're in at the moment. We're happy that this is happening, but we're both mourning a little bit. She's mourning this evolution of her body that she never wanted. And I'm mourning watching her, something so close that I can't have. It's a really interesting dynamic with us where we're happy but also quite sad. And we're just rolling with it and talking a lot about it."**

Communication is the key that has kept them together and connected.

> **"Every time the baby kicks, she's like, 'This feels gross.' And I'm like, 'Oh, I wish I could feel that. Tell me what it feels like.' She goes, 'It feels like a trapped fart. Look at my boobs, they're massive! It's disgusting.' But I'm looking at her thinking, 'I wish this was happening to me.' So yeah, it's a really alternate universe that we're living in."**

Crystal and Kate plan to have their baby in Moree, the closest hospital to their home. Everyone in their community is aware of Kate's cancer journey and so many have shown incredible support. And the community is now looking out for Crystal during her pregnancy.

Kate realises what an incredible sacrifice her amazing wife has made.

> **"It's a huge gift. It is the biggest gift of love. You only have to meet her for five minutes to determine that this is not her. This was not her life plan."**

One thing the couple has worked out is that Kate is the better patient and Crystal is the better nurse. When the roles were reversed and Crystal had two weeks of morning sickness, Kate described her wife as a horrendous patient who was much better at being a nurse!

Kate continues her recovery and search for effective treatment of her current conditions—she now has lymphoedema in her leg and groin and also a pain in her hip. It immediately made her think that the cancer had returned, but her doctor diagnosed a bone fracture from the radiation.

"Since the moment I had gluten intolerance to what I have now, I've learnt that no one is going to look after you the way that you look after yourself. You've got to create that team of people and you've got to find services that are near you. It's a lot of trial and error and a lot of money spent but you need to find the people who are going to help you."

As they wait for their baby to arrive, Kate is back doing part-time desk work and, because she has the time, she has started a diploma of counselling. She has also expanded her creative outlet of beading into a business called The Blissful Thistle. Named after her glamorous Scottish grandma, Kate makes beautiful beaded bracelets that are not only gorgeous pieces of jewellery, but they also gift the wearer with the healing energy of the crystal beads.

Through her business and Instagram account, Kate has connected with many women, sharing her experience and knowledge and offering hope, the way that only someone who has walked the walk, can.

"We are just like everyone else. Except for the whole cancer and egg swap. That's a little bit different. But we're just making a family in whatever way we can, with the options that we had."

PS. On the first of August, Crystal and Kate's miracle was born—Zoe is a gorgeous and healthy baby girl. Congratulations to the new mums!

3

NERIDA

- Polycystic Ovary Syndrome (PCOS)*
- Haemorrhagic Ovarian Cyst*
- Gestational Diabetes
- Chloé, aged one, Hip Dysplasia*, Biliary Atresia*

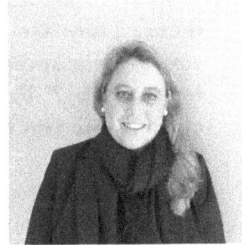

When Nerida and Angus met at Orange Agricultural College, neither of them imagined that their lives would converge again almost two decades later. After graduation, their careers took them on different paths with Nerida moving to Sydney to take up a career in real estate then in travel.

An opportunity to open a new Flight Centre store in Orange took Nerida back to her hometown. She successfully established the new business and then continued her career in travel in Sydney, working for Malaysian Airlines and Scenic Tours over a period of 10 years.

Even though she had always held the dream of getting married and having children, by the time she was in her early thirties, Nerida had not yet met the right man and she was starting to wonder if it was going to happen.

When she was 33, Nerida was forced to think seriously about her plans to have children. Abdominal pain led to a diagnosis of PCOS when tests showed a large cyst on her ovary was haemorrhaging. The cyst had attached itself to her bowel and spine and required a complex surgery to remove it.

Because PCOS is a hormonal issue, it can lead to difficulties with falling pregnant. This medical condition added another obstacle to Nerida's ability to have children and influenced her thoughts about the future.

"I am the youngest of four and have always wanted children. I thought that if I don't have children by the time I am 35 then I'm going to freeze my eggs. It was a done deal in my head."

Nerida's doctor talked her through the process of harvesting eggs, outlining the costs as well as the realistic chances of her eggs becoming successful embryos. He was frank in his opinion, saying, "You might spend all this money and you may get two or three eggs. And those two or three eggs may not take, and you've spent a fortune."

His opinion was blunt, causing Nerida to think long and hard about her situation. It seemed more and more likely that motherhood was not going to happen for her.

"I have 10 nieces and nephews. I've put my heart and soul into them. They are my world and I absolutely adore them. The youngest is seven and they asked me, 'When are you going to have a baby?' I'm like, 'There is no such thing as immaculate conception. Got to find a man.'"

Nerida shares an especially close relationship with her sister's children. Their mother had suffered from alcoholism which had required extended periods away at rehabilitation. Nerida became their 'other mum', often helping her parents take care of them.

With these beautiful children in her life, Nerida wondered if they were enough, if perhaps somehow, that was the way it was meant to be and that she should be grateful for what she had.

"I got to thinking, 'It's not going to happen. I'm too old now. I'm not going to find somebody.' I just gave up and decided to travel."

Taking advantage of working in the travel industry, Nerida accepted every opportunity to visit spectacular places around the world, from the exotic luxury of the Maldives to the history and culture of Cambodia.

In between her adventures, Nerida's eldest sister suggested she see a doctor who had helped some her of friends with hormone issues. Called an integrative doctor, the practitioner is a qualified GP who also focuses on preventative medicine and nutrition in a more holistic approach to treating patients. At the time, Nerida thought it was a good idea because she had been feeling lacklustre and lethargic.

"I met with her and she said to me, 'With your hormones and polycystic ovaries, get off the contraception.'"

Nerida was using contraception originally prescribed to regulate her erratic periods. She agreed with the treatment plan, thinking she should have done it earlier because she had already been told that falling pregnant was highly unlikely.

Between helping out with family, running her own travel agency and travelling extensively, Nerida was keeping busy, happily living the life she had chosen. But all of that was about to change.

It took the modern wonder of social media for Nerida and Angus to cross paths. They started dating during a particularly busy time for Nerida. She had agreed to house-sit for a friend in Sydney and, true to her decision to spend her money on travel, she had five trips lined up that year.

Just before her trip to the Maldives, Nerida went to her doctor for some general blood tests. She mentioned to her doctor that her period had not come. Since she had stopped contraception under medical advice, Nerida had expected her periods to be erratic so the fact that they were not regular was no surprise. The doctor thought it would be a good idea to check for pregnancy and said he would add that test to the pathology.

"When I rang him for the results he said, 'Your blood tests are fine.' And I said, 'Oh, and the pregnancy result?' And he said, 'Oh, the pregnancy. No, that's negative.'"

Nerida jumped on the plane to the Maldives and when she returned, she only had a few days at home before heading off to Hawaii with a friend. While away, Nerida had breast and abdominal pain which persisted and despite the test results, her friend insisted that she was pregnant.

Once home, she returned to her doctor and asked for an ultrasound.

"I was told that I wasn't pregnant, so I thought I had another cyst on my ovary. That's why my period was all out of whack. I just thought it was a repeat of that."

Thinking that she was going for the routine ultrasound of a cyst, Nerida went on her own. The sonographer started looking around and asked about the negative-for-pregnancy blood test.

"She said, 'Well, you've got a little gestation sac there with a heartbeat.' And I just burst into tears and said, 'What?' She said, 'You're about eight weeks and three days.' I was shocked. I was absolutely blown away."

The news was extraordinary, especially when Nerida had been told definitively by her doctor that she was not pregnant. Angus and Nerida had so much to consider and it forced them to discuss subjects that usually do not arise until a relationship is much more established.

"It wasn't something that we had planned. It wasn't this elation. It was fear. There were tears. There was uncertainty. My family was thrilled for me. They said things like, 'Oh, my gosh, you're having a baby, finally. You're going to have your own little one. You've done so much for all your nieces and nephews. It's now your turn.' Everyone was over the moon."

From the moment I met Angus and Nerida, it was obvious that they communicate honestly and openly with each other. There is no doubt that their willingness to hear and understand each other's feelings contributed to their capacity to navigate what was to come.

The couple was unified in their decision to proceed with the pregnancy. Nerida firmly believed, "If it's meant to be, it's meant to be." One thing that did concern them was the doctor's original blood test result. They later asked their obstetrician to go through the pathology records to check exactly what had been tested and the inquiry revealed that the doctor had actually made a mistake—the pregnancy test was never requested.

"It was really bad on his behalf. I did two overseas trips. I was getting ready to go to Zimbabwe. I was having all my vaccinations to get ready for that trip and I found out that I had one of the vaccines that you're not meant to have when you're pregnant. If the doctor hadn't told me a lie, I would have known not to have it."

The thought that she had perhaps harmed her baby with the vaccine was something that worried Nerida throughout her pregnancy, even though she knew that she had only been acting on the advice she had been given. Fortunately, she had not yet had her vaccination for malaria for her next trip, which would also not have been advised for pregnant women. Nerida contacted the Health Department's Communicable Disease Authority and they recommended an alternative that was safe for pregnancy.

"I was nervous about taking it, thinking that they weren't 100% on it. I'd already had this other vaccination. All of this plays on your mind."

Nerida also struggled with her own feelings. She had removed children from her future plans, and this meant that the money she would otherwise have saved for a house, mortgage, children and their education, had been hers to spend as she pleased. Now, that picture had been flipped around completely. She was 38 years old, her window for having children was closing, this pregnancy was likely her only chance to have her own child, and yet she felt completely unprepared emotionally, physically and financially.

Despite the nervousness she felt throughout her pregnancy, Nerida soon started feeling excited. Just before she went to Zimbabwe, she attended her first obstetric appointment. PCOS made her a likely candidate for gestational diabetes and the doctor suggested that she probably already had it. As soon as she returned from her trip, Nerida went for a Glucose Tolerance Test (GTT)* and it came back positive at only 10 weeks' gestation.

Further testing suggested that she possibly had Type 2 Diabetes* prior to pregnancy, but this has now been shown not to be the case. Either way, it was important that she see an endocrinologist*. The couple were fortunate to find a specialist who deals specifically with diabetes and pregnancy and this doctor managed her condition throughout. She prescribed Nerida with a medication called Metformin* along with a very strict diet.

"It's very important to have carbs for the development of the foetus. I was trying to get my head around a whole new diet and medication."

Nerida tested her blood sugar four times a day and charted her results. That report was sent to the endocrinologist every day and they would wait for a reply with adjustments to the dosage of her medication. With the doctor located in Sydney and the couple some 250km away in Orange, the majority of their appointments were via Skype.

A few weeks later, the couple attended their 13-week scan. Considered a high-risk pregnancy due to her age and gestational diabetes, they also had the Nuchal Translucency* scan to check for Down Syndrome* and they were pleased to receive a negative result. They also had the Harmony* blood test to check for chromosomal issues and this yielded an inconclusive result. Thankfully, a second Harmony test also confirmed the baby was completely healthy.

The couple had not made a conscious decision not to find out the sex of the baby, but Nerida accidentally stumbled upon the information.

> **"I asked one of the GPs if I could have a copy of the Harmony test so I could see what it said. I'm walking down the hallway and went, 'Ahhhhh!' My baby is a girl. You can't unsee that."**

Nerida worked hard to take care of herself and to be in the best possible health for her baby. She quit smoking and stuck to the strict diet and medication regime. Nerida also required Anti D injections* due to her A negative blood type, and insulin injections from around 28 weeks.

As her due date approached, the obstetrician had hoped that the baby would turn from the breech position, the way she had been since the six-month mark. The doctor and the endocrinologist tussled over the baby's delivery date. The obstetrician was hesitant to let the baby go full-term and the endocrinologist wanting the baby to stay in as long as possible. They eventually settled on 38 weeks.

At 36 weeks and five days, the doctor asked them to come in to check the baby's position. Sure enough, she was still breech. The obstetrician began talking to the couple about spinning the baby and the risks involved.

> **"I didn't care how she came out. Of course, you always want to think that you can have a baby naturally, but a lot of things weren't on my side. I was not fazed at whether it was going to be an epidural or a caesarean, I just wanted the doctor to get us through this alive."**

Nerida's blood pressure was high. Her medical team were concerned and decided to keep her overnight for observation. They laid out a plan to monitor her over the weekend, then with all going well, they would give her a steroid injection the following Tuesday and Wednesday with the intention of starting induction on the Thursday. Because the baby would be born premature at 37 weeks, the steroid injections were provided to give a helping hand to the baby's lungs.

Over the weekend, Nerida's blood pressure continued to rise, so they connected her to an electrocardiograph*.

> **"The paper ended up going for miles because she wasn't a very active baby. Throughout the whole pregnancy, I could barely feel her, she didn't move much. They had me on the trace for about three or four hours and they were looking for all these accelerations and there just weren't any there.**

My blood pressure was 210/110. They called my midwife and she talked to the head midwife who said, 'Sorry, this is protocol. I'm going to have to hit it.' So they hit the emergency button and I freaked out!"

The room instantly filled with medical staff prepping her for an emergency caesarean. Nerida was swabbed, fitted with a cannula and injected with medication to lower her blood pressure. As they swarmed around her, Nerida insisted she was fine. She was actually more concerned about a large group of her clients who were stuck in Buenos Aires airport due to a workers' strike.

As their travel agent, Nerida needed to contact a company based in Singapore to arrange new e-tickets and she was still on the phone making arrangements while they wheeled her down to theatre. She was so engrossed in fixing the problem that she didn't fully realise the serious nature of her personal situation.

Angus received the emergency call at work and rushed straight to the hospital. He met Nerida in her room before theatre and then stayed in a waiting bay while Nerida was prepped. The anaesthetist was in the process of giving Nerida a spinal block when they all heard the sound of another emergency button being pushed in the birthing suite. That woman had already had her epidural so it was decided that she would jump the queue and go in first. The anaesthetist took the needle out of Nerida and went into theatre with the other woman.

The heightened chaos suddenly vanished as quickly as it had begun, and as there was a pause in proceedings, Angus was called from the waiting bay and the couple found themselves alone in a waiting room.

"I think I went into shock then because it just kind of dawned on me what the hell was going on because I'd finally got my tickets off to Buenos Aires. I started to shiver and shake, and they covered me with all these hot blankets."

After waiting for about half an hour, it was time to proceed, The serendipity of the delay was that it allowed enough time for their own obstetrician to arrive in time to deliver their baby. The other plus was then having the services of the head anaesthetist who handled that part of the operation beautifully.

Chloé arrived into the world at 5.17pm and had a beautiful cuddle on Nerida's chest for a few minutes before the staff whisked her off to the Neonatal Intensive Care Unit (NICU)*.

From her bloods, the medical staff could see that Chloé's sugars were below acceptable levels. This was a possibility that the couple had been prepared for due to the presence of gestational diabetes. Angus went with their baby while Nerida was taken to recovery.

"They put a cannula into Chloé with that first blood test and it was in the range where they had to go to higher authorities," said Angus. "They used it to give her a little bit of glucose."

The newborn stabilised but they still kept her in the NICU. Meanwhile, Nerida was in recovery experiencing the side effects of the anaesthetic.

"It was wild itchiness. As the anaesthetic started to wear off, my arms and back were so itchy. The recovery nurse was saying please don't itch. I was thinking, 'I'm not interested in what you have to say right now!'"

Once she was back in the ward, Nerida desperately wanted to see her baby. Mothers who are not walking are generally not allowed in NICU as they do not have any equipment to resuscitate adults. There was no way Nerida could walk so one of the nurses wheeled her in on her bed. Nerida saw her baby, but the effort made her faint and she collapsed on the bed.

The next day, a NICU nurse told the couple that they were going to do a test because Chloé had a little jaundice. They used a non-invasive transcutaneous bilirubinometer* and plotted the results. Her readings showed that Chloé's results were slightly in the range of requiring phototherapy so they put her into light therapy and also took a blood sample for analysis.

To facilitate feeding, Chloé was fitted with a Nasogastric Tube (NGT)* and this method was used to deliver Nerida's colostrum*.

"I couldn't feed her from the start because she was still in NICU and I couldn't get to her. I couldn't walk and was very unsteady for a while. The surgery really knocked me around."

Angus and Nerida's concerns for Chloé's health was based on the understanding that she had jaundice, a common occurrence in newborns, that would be resolved after a few days under lights. Up to this point, they had no idea that their daughter had more serious issues.

Two days after her birth, Nerida recovered her mobility sufficiently to walk and with Angus's assistance, they went to see Chloé in the NICU. As they entered, a paediatrician asked to have a chat.

> **"She told us they had just been talking to Westmead Children's Hospital. I nearly collapsed on the floor. They sat me down and the doctor started talking. I said to her, 'I can't listen to this. It's making me really uptight.' She had no bedside manner."**

Angus was equally shocked.

> **"We didn't have any pre-curser to this," confirmed Angus. "We didn't even know that the hospital had been talking to Westmead and it seemed like they'd been talking to them about it for at least a day."**

Chloé's blood had been sent for the split bilirubin blood test* that checks for the ratio of conjugated and unconjugated bilirubin. The total levels were dangerously high, but the real concern was the level of the conjugated bilirubin, the part that does not respond to light therapy. It is an indicator of a variety of other more serious issues and led one of the paediatricians to say, "We're not sure what's going on. We think that she might not have a gall bladder."

Angus doubted this diagnosis because he was sure that a gallbladder had been sighted on one of Chloé's previous scans. There appeared to be lots of questions and unknowns and no definite answers or solutions.

> **"They told us we may have to be airlifted to Westmead, but we had to wait until we could have another ultrasound and that couldn't be done until the next day. When you've had as many ultrasounds as we've had, you think you're home and hosed. But when you hear she's got no gallbladder, you think, 'Why is this all happening? I don't understand.'"**

The following morning, the sonographer found that Chloé actually did have a gallbladder, but that there appeared to be a restriction or blockage in the main bile duct between her liver and intestine. The medical team did more tests, sending the results to Westmead in their effort to correctly diagnose the problem.

By the end of the day, the resident paediatrician gave the couple a variety of possible causes. They could not get a full image of the bile ducts through ultrasound, but from what they could see, it looked like a Choledochal cyst* had formed outside the bile duct. If that was the case, Chloé would require a small procedure to either drain or remove the cyst and there was a good chance that the flow from her liver to her intestine would return. The other very unlikely possibility was a rare disease called biliary atresia, where the bile flow is blocked causing damage to the liver.

"We were told she didn't have it, but we googled it anyway. It became our biggest fear, but at the time we said, 'Thank god she doesn't have it.'"

The couple was told that there was no need to worry because they were fairly sure it was a cyst and that it was something they could easily treat. The doctor also advised that just to be sure, Chloé's case would be reviewed at a multidisciplinary meeting at Westmead Hospital the following Wednesday. In the meantime, he told them to go home.

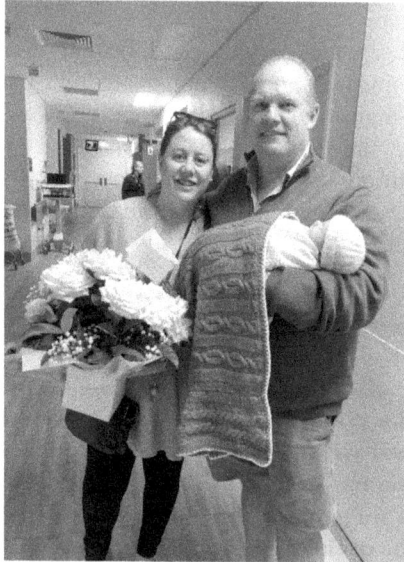

Nerida and Angus taking Chloe home from Orange Hospital

With great trepidation, the new parents took their baby home. Hoping for clarification on Chloé's prognosis, Nerida sought advice from a long-time family friend who was a retired paediatrician.

"I asked, 'What does the cyst mean? Is it day surgery?' He said that because babies are so tiny, we would probably be in for at least 10 days. Oh my god, it was huge. Just a little blockage could cause two weeks in Westmead."

A few days later, Nerida received a call to say that Chloé definitely had a problem and that there was a lot to discuss, but they would not do it over the phone. It was a Tuesday, exactly one week after Chloé was born, and the doctors asked them to come in on Wednesday afternoon.

The next 24-hour period was intolerable. Knowing that there was something wrong with their baby but with no information on what it was, left Nerida and Angus in a frustrating and upsetting limbo that filled them with dread.

When they arrived at the hospital the following day, the couple was met by their paediatrician, the registrar and the nurse unit manager. Nerida is thankful for the kindness of their paediatrician whose gentle approach helped them to take in the information. They were told that at that point, they believed that Chloé had biliary atresia.

"I just burst into tears. I was uncontrollable. It was a lot of information. They were very slow, very methodical and said that they don't know how it was caused. They don't know if it happens in utero* or if it happens straight after birth. They really don't know what causes it and that's the biggest mystery. I was an absolute mess, devastated to hear the news. It was just a nightmare."

The paediatrician advised that further tests were required to confirm their daughter's diagnosis. They needed to work out exactly where Chloé's bile flow was blocked to determine what needed to be done.

Realising the enormity of the situation and complexity of the disease, the doctor recommended that they take one step at a time, focussing on each part of the process rather than panicking about what might happen down the track. It was sound advice, but difficult to action.

Chloé was expected at Westmead on the following Tuesday. Preparing for their trip to the hospital was so hard. With no idea how of long they might be there and the emotional stress of what their baby was about to face, the couple felt the strain of packing and leaving their home and driving four hours to the Children's Hospital.

On Tuesday morning, doctors began the first test, a DISIDA* scan to examine the gallbladder and hepatobiliary* system with a radioactive trace. The results confirmed that there was no flow of bile and they were informed that they would need to move on to the next stage with a test called a cholangiogram*.

This required surgery to conduct a physical examination of the organs. A tracer dye was injected directly into the gallbladder and bile ducts and then scanned by fluoroscopy* (x-ray video) so that surgeons could watch in real time to see whether or not the tracer flowed through the bile ducts.

The doctors suggested that there could be a faint chance that a flush of the bile ducts with saline could restore flow, but if this did not work, they would have to proceed with a Kasai* procedure that surgically bypasses the blocked ducts to allow the bile to drain from the liver to the intestine.

With the cholangiogram scheduled for the following Monday, Nerida and Angus had the choice of going home and returning but due to the distance between hospital and home as well as how incredibly hard it was to start the initial journey to Westmead earlier that week, they decided to stay.

One day shy of three weeks old, Chloé was prepared for the cholangiogram. It was a long and emotional morning—Angus and Nerida had to deal with their own anxiety while consoling their fasting baby. There were delays in operating time and it was frustrating to see other children being admitted more quickly than they were. After the pre-operation checks, it was heart-wrenching to hand Chloé over to the anaesthetist.

> **"Would it be a short operation with Chloé given the all clear, or a much longer operation with greater risk and an uncertain outcome? We just paced back and forth in the hospital and went to the NICU area where they said they would bring her.**
>
> **They were a couple of hours into the operation when they called Angus and confirmed it was biliary atresia and there was no flow, so they were going to proceed with the Kasai procedure."**

Chloé's gallbladder was quite small, and the walls of her gallbladder were very thick, but the main problem was that there was a blockage preventing the bile from getting from the liver to her small intestine. The procedure involved removing her gallbladder and the damaged and blocked ducts between her liver and intestine and trimming the outer layer of her liver to expose fresh ducts underneath. They then took a piece of her small intestine and connected her liver directly to her intestine. After six hours, Chloé finally emerged from theatre.

> **"She came back to NICU and she was hooked up to everything under the sun and it was awful. It was the most horrific thing to see my little baby like that."**

The surgeon reassured the worried parents that their baby was stable and that the surgery was a great success. They had expected the liver to show cirrhosis and scarring but it was pink and healthy. The doctor informed them that they would know how well the Kasai had worked within around three months.

Chloé steadily improved from her operation in NICU. Nerida laughed as she showed me pictures of her daughter's poo, explaining that if it was a white, pasty colour, then that was an indicator that the bile was not getting through to the intestine. The day her poo was that normal green, mustard colour that all parents know too well, was a cause for celebration!

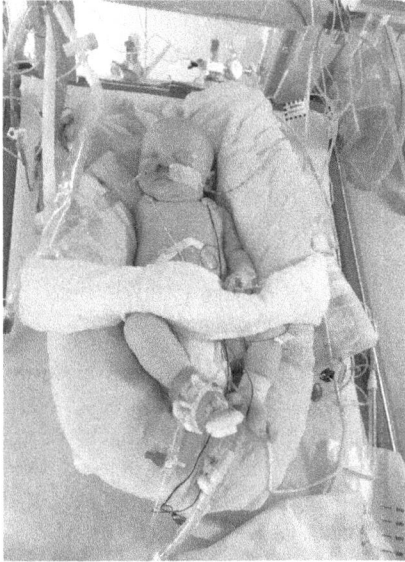

Chloé in NICU

After a month in recovery, Chloé was finally allowed to go home. Upon discharge, the medical staff spoke in strong terms about the dangers of infection and warned them to keep their baby away from shops and busy places with lots of people. Any type of infection could be devastating for Chloé, even a cold could be the start of something much worse.

At home, the couple instigated common sense practices to keep Chloé's environment as healthy as possible. Visitors were asked to wash their hands or use sanitiser, and if they were sick, they needed to keep their distance. They also consciously reduced the chemicals in their home and chose more natural alternatives.

Four weeks post-surgery, Nerida and Angus returned with Chloé to Westmead for her check-up. The doctors were pleased to see her progress and admitted that they had not expected such good results.

"She's actually kind of a miracle. Even the doctors are shocked at how well she's doing. The surgeon actually said that he

didn't think it was going to work. He thought the Kasai would fail and he wasn't confident in her when she was discharged."

The surgeons were satisfied that the operation had proceeded well but they were uncertain as to what the overall outcome would be. Normally, if the Kasai fails, it will do so in the first three months and the baby will be sick and deteriorate. At that point, there is no option but a liver transplant. Angus informed me that around 30% of babies with biliary atresia will need a transplant before the age of two, and that 80% will require a liver transplant at some point in their life.

Not only do they need to prepare for this likely outcome, but Nerida and Angus also have to help Chloé deal with the constant threat of cholangitis* due to the fact that bacteria from her bowel can flow back to her liver. One of the first symptoms is a fever, and if this occurs, they take Chloé directly to hospital where she is administered IV antibiotics for 48 hours because if the cholangitis gets into the liver, it takes hold and can cause life-threatening damage.

Even if her elevated temperature is caused by something as simple as teething, a cold or any relatively trivial illness, Nerida and Angus are unable to take the usual parental approach of giving Chloé some medication and waiting to see what develops. Due to the need for immediate treatment just in case she has cholangitis, they need to attend hospital promptly, armed with a rapid treatment plan and instant admission instructions from Westmead so that antibiotic treatment can be commenced while pathology testing is underway.

To date Chloé has only had to go through this once. She takes various medications and supplements and is defying all expectations. Angus and Nerida are taking a protective yet practical approach in their mission to create the best possible future for their daughter.

"At first, we envisaged that we'd be constantly in hospital with every single sniffle or fever, but that hasn't happened," said Angus. "We're transitioning from completely wrapping her in a bubble to the next stage where she's now rolling.

She's on the floor, we've got a dog in the house and we're now at the stage of trying to do natural immunisation against getting sick because she might get really sick down the track and need a transplant which will compromise her immune system. The worst didn't happen so now we actually need to rethink and prepare her to get ready for life."

The couple have developed a collaborative relationship with Chloé's medical team. At her post-birth discharge examination, the doctor noticed a click in Chloé's hip and referred her for a hip ultrasound to be conducted at 12 weeks from her due date. She was diagnosed with hip dysplasia and was fitted with a brace to help her hip develop normally. The initial six week period was extended for a further 12 weeks during which time Chloé wore the brace 24 hours a day for the first two months, then gradually reduced the time to eight hours a day by the fifth month after which time she no longer needed it.

For a baby going through all of this trauma, it would be reasonable to expect her to be unsettled or sleepless, but Chloé is neither—she is a delightfully calm and happy baby who has slept through the night since she was seven weeks old!

During her post-operation recovery period at Westmead, Chloé had several additional scans due to the fact that biliary atresia can occur in conjunction with other internal organ defects. One of these was a heart echo cardiogram* which revealed a heart murmur, indicating a patent foramen ovale* (hole in the heart) and pulmonary stenosis*.

This raised concerns with the doctors that Chloé could also have Allagille Syndrome* and she underwent a specific test to check if any genetic markers were present. Those tests came back clear and a later visit to a cardiologist at six months of age and further scans of her heart confirmed that the problem has now resolved itself.

First-time motherhood is a challenging new experience for every woman, but Nerida's came with layers of complexity. I asked her how she handled those first few months with Chloé.

> **"It's an emotional thing. You can't help but be emotional, but I think you need to be rational. Friends and family would say, 'Have a glass of wine and relax.' I would say no because I needed to be on my best game. I needed to be focussed. I needed to understand what was going on. I didn't get carried away with Googling but got the facts from the doctors. I had to stay strong for my little baby and keep my head on straight."**

Angus is the first to praise Nerida for the amazing job she has done in nurturing Chloé. He shared how careful she was with her diet and health throughout the pregnancy. Despite there being no medical evidence that Chloé's health issues were a result of anything she had done during pregnancy, Nerida still had a hard time coming to terms with it.

"One of the hardest things to reconcile was the tremendous guilt that Nerida felt about whether or not it was something she had done," shared Angus. "Whether it could be traced back to activities of her health, that extra glass of wine at the wrong time or something she ate or some stress in her body."

Nerida wonders how things might have been different if she had known she was pregnant before her trips. That knowledge would have stopped her from having the travel vaccine and likely caused her to cancel her trip.

"I didn't know that I was pregnant. We've talked about it time and time again. They have no idea why it happened. What's helped me is time, I think, and understanding that it's the way that it is. There was no linkage. So yeah, I certainly went through all that, but now I just love her and I just adore her. She's just the best thing."

A trauma with a child, especially a baby, is challenging in any circumstances but for Nerida and Angus, they were also navigating a new relationship. I asked the couple how they coped during the trauma of the past year.

"We're very open with our communication. We talk about our fears, our joys, our wins. We talk about everything and at least we know where we're both mentally sitting at that point so we can be considerate and say, 'Right, you're not having a great day because you're stressed and I'm not having a great day because I've been busy.' But you support each other and communicate because it's critical."

Angus agreed that communication is the key.

"We have been together, focussed on her well-being and I think that has helped. It has meant that we can talk things through and we're not afraid to show our distress with stuff for her and we talk about it."

Angus and Nerida have no illusions about the road ahead. Chloé has a disease that will impact her for the rest of her life.

"She's super special and she's just that little bit extra special because she does have a lifelong disease. It's not something she's going to get over. It's forever. Even if she keeps her native

liver, she can never have a drink. She won't be able to do anything that's going to affect her liver."

Chloé will always have to do regular blood work and liver function tests. She will have challenges and bouts of cholangitis. She will likely need a liver transplant and that will require anti-rejection medication for the rest of her life. She may have more than one transplant. She will need to manage her lifestyle to reduce strain on her liver, even to the point of not being able to take over the counter pain medication. They are aware and prepared for what could happen but hopeful for a different outcome.

"Hope is a good thing," said Angus. "We did a lot of worst-case scenarios, what ifs, and we would never dream of being in a position to have this good an outcome. We've had so many moments thinking that this is going to be the beginning of the end and it hasn't happened."

Biliary Atresia is such a rare disease with only 1 in 8,000 to 1 in 18,000 babies affected depending on ethnicity. Nerida and Angus are now strong advocates for the split bilirubin test and support the recommendations of medical experts to conduct this test on all infants showing signs of jaundice two to three weeks after birth.

It is important to correctly diagnose a baby before six weeks of age otherwise it may be too late for the Kasai procedure that saved Chloé. Babies who are not diagnosed in time can suffer significant liver damage and their only hope is a liver transplant.

The couple's understanding of the transplant process has also driven their support of organ donation. They learned that there is a constant shortage of donors and that becoming a donor really is a lifesaving decision. An adult liver can be separated into two parts, so an adult liver donor can save the life of both an adult and a baby or child.

The availability of donor organs is vitally important because babies on the transplant list are ordered in priority of need. The most critical baby is put to the top of the list and sadly, some babies do not make it.

As Chloé approaches her first birthday, she is kicking goals and thriving. Her physical strength and delightful temperament are already having a positive impact on her life and all of those around her. There is no doubt that Chloe's future is bright in the capable hands of her parents.

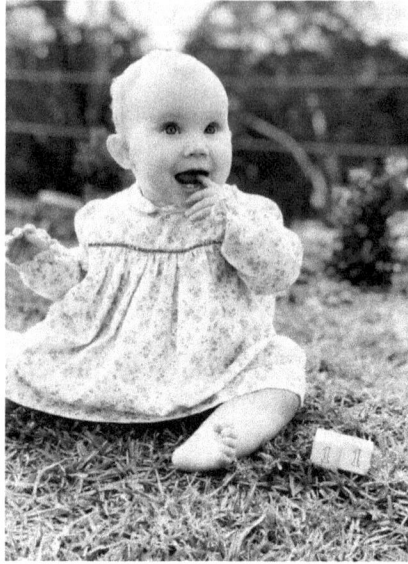

Chloé at 10 months

"We thought our life would be turned on its head. We thought that by this point in time we would be down at Westmead for months doing a transplant but we're not there yet and you know what, I just take every good day as a good day. I say that quote often. 'Today's a good day. Let's not worry about tomorrow, just enjoy today.' We don't know what will happen next week or next month and we're not going to sit here and think it's all doom and gloom. You've got to be positive."

4

MELINDA

- 12 Pregnancies
- Pre-eclampsia*
- Angel baby* Declan
- HELLP Syndrome*
- Rainbow baby Hudson, aged four
- Intrauterine Insemination (IUI)*
- Three cycles of IVF

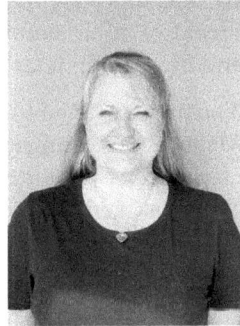

For as far back as she can remember, Melinda has always wanted to be a mum. She recalls a childhood spent happily playing with dolls with her sister and playing mother to her younger brother who arrived when she was eight years old. By the time she was 13, Melinda was already trusted to babysit children and she was even nanny to a newborn!

Melinda's love of children influenced her decision to become a primary school teacher, a career she has enjoyed for more than 20 years. She was thrilled to get married at 22, full of hope and the expectation of having her own large family. This was not to be—Melinda found herself divorced and single at 25, feeling like "used trash".

Undeterred, Melinda refused to give up on her dream to have children. The problem was finding the right man to share her vision. The year was 2002 and she decided to try out the new online dating sites.

"Back then, it was kind of an uncool way to meet someone. You would meet them on the internet, but you would tell people

that you met somewhere else. It was different, now it's just normal."

Melinda met 'hundreds of weirdos' as she trawled through the internet sites for eight years. By that time, she'd become quite savvy regarding what to look for in a potential date's profile. In 2010, a guy named Lincoln was interested in Melinda, but she was instantly wary because he had not uploaded a photo. Within 10 seconds of asking for one, it was uploaded, and the pair began chatting. Three weeks later they met face to face.

"He was nice, but I gave him a really hard time because I'd been through the wringer with all these other losers."

She had become so jaded with bad dates that she nearly missed the good one! Friends encouraged her to give Lincoln a decent chance and she finally arranged a real date and found that she liked him. They started dating and in 2013 were married.

By that time, Melinda was 35 and her biological clock was ticking. Her dream of a big family meant that they needed to get started right away and five months later, they discovered they were pregnant!

The first few months of pregnancy were fairly routine. In hindsight, Melinda remembers the blissful naivety of her straightforward expectations: a woman gets pregnant, the embryo grows, after 40 weeks it comes out and then you have a baby in your arms.

At 20 weeks, a dramatic accident changed everything. Melinda attended a baseball game with her father, brother and Lincoln and they were seated up in the stands. During a break in the game, all of the spectators were invited to stand up for the chance to catch a baseball and win a prize. Melinda stood, looked up at her brother and lost her balance. She found herself flying through the air over the rows of seats and then landed in the first row of their tier after desperately grabbing the railing because she knew there was a steep drop on the other side.

"It was like slow motion. As I was flying, I knew I had to grab that bar because if I didn't, I was going over. I had this, 'Oh my god, I have to stop myself' moment before crashing onto the seats. I couldn't breathe and I was in panic mode that I'd hurt my baby."

Melinda was rushed to hospital in an ambulance. Thankfully, mother and baby were fine. At the time, she was relieved, but in her mind, Melinda marks this event as perhaps the start of their pregnancy problems.

By 24 weeks, Melinda's health began to seriously deteriorate, and she was experiencing chronic high blood pressure. Her doctors tried various ways to control it, but nothing worked.

"I didn't feel well. I didn't feel like myself. I had no energy. I was always tired, but people say that's part of pregnancy. If I was doing it all again, I would do it differently. Listening to your body is an instinct and I should have trusted it."

Melinda's obstetrician went on holidays and because she was at risk of developing pre-eclampsia*, she needed daily medical attention and was passed from doctor to doctor. When her own specialist returned, he looked at Melinda's blood tests and told her to admit herself to hospital the following day, prescribing bed rest until the baby was born. She was only 26 weeks pregnant.

"Well, I was distraught. 14 weeks in a hospital bed. Now if someone had said to me that if I didn't do it, I would lose my baby, then I most certainly would have done it without a question. But the thought of losing my baby didn't cross my mind."

The first night in hospital, alone in the dark, Melinda cried all night. She did not want to be there. She never imagined her pregnancy developing this way. Her frustration increased further when they would not allow her to walk, not even to go to the toilet! Melinda felt that the precautions were ridiculous and all she wanted to do was to go home.

The next day, Lincoln returned to the hospital with the items required for Melinda's long stay, arriving in time to accompany her to a scheduled ultrasound to measure the baby. With her blood pressure a major issue, the plan was to deliver the baby as soon as a viable weight was achieved.

"I wanted to see how heavy the baby was. If I was to go through this all again, I needed to look at the heartbeat first."

A young girl was conducting the scan. She moved the wand here and there while Melinda look intently at the screen trying to see the weight of the baby. Eventually, the sonographer excused herself and then returned with an older woman who was the radiographer and practice owner. The woman looked at the screen and said eight words, "There is no heartbeat —shut off the machine," before immediately exiting the room.

"I'm thinking, 'Don't shut off the machine! I haven't seen how heavy it is yet. I need to know how heavy this baby is.' It didn't register to me. Lincoln was crying as he had comprehended what we were told but for me, the whole world stopped because I wasn't seeing what I needed to see."

Melinda was in complete denial. She could not believe what she had been told. It had to be a mistake. She just could not comprehend that her baby was gone.

Amidst all the pain and confusion, Melinda was told that she would be put into labour that night. The news was shocking—if the baby was gone, she just wanted it taken out. The midwife explained that she needed to go into natural labour, and it was then that the impact of her situation really hit her.

Shortly after, Melinda's mother, sister and nephew popped in for a visit, having no knowledge of what had just transpired.

"I announced that I had just lost the baby and that was it, everyone was bawling. I will never forget it. It was a pain that I still can't describe…the pain of losing my beautiful baby."

Melinda was induced at 9:30pm and endured 16 hours of labour. Not only was it physically painful, but it was emotional torture. She knew she was giving birth to someone who was never going to come home with her—going through all this agony for a baby that wasn't breathing.

At the 14-hour mark, Melinda was in so much pain that she could not sit up. The doctor came in to administer an epidural and said, "For god's sake, sit up straight - didn't you listen at your classes?" Melinda screamed, "I can't." Lincoln then said, "We didn't make it far enough to get to them," and somehow through anger and exhaustion, Melinda straightened up for the injection to be administered.

"I felt like everyone was mean. My world was destroyed right there and then. This doctor was awful to me, the person at the ultrasound was awful. There was no empathy."

Melinda was asked if she wanted to hold the baby when it was born. She said no. Death was something she had never dealt with before and there was no way she was going to hold a dead baby.

After her final push, Declan Noah Parker slipped into the world silently. The doctor told her it was a boy. At that moment, Melinda's maternal instincts kicked in and she felt an overwhelming desperation to hold her baby because in that instant, he was no longer just a baby—he was her beautiful baby boy.

The caring midwives wrapped Declan in a blanket and placed him in Melinda's arms. It looked like a typical childbirth scene until her vital signs became unstable. Melinda had a rare condition called HELLP Syndrome, causing the red cells in her blood to break down.

At this point, Lincoln had to deal with even more trauma. He had just lost his son, and now he was facing the possibility of losing his wife.

The medical team was eventually able to stabilise Melinda, but they insisted that she stay in hospital for a few days to fully recover as her organs were not functioning properly. She was given her own room with Declan in a crib beside her, just like any other baby. The only problem was that the only available room was in the delivery ward.

"They were long nights. There was just Lincoln, Declan and me. All night, all we heard were people pushing, people screaming, people running, babies crying. And right beside us in our crib was ours that was never going to cry."

Despite the difficulty of their surroundings, Melinda and Lincoln were both grateful for the time together. It allowed them to have the family and one friend come to visit and meet Declan. He was only 400 grams but looked just like his daddy. A photographer came to take photos and they were able to record their treasured moments, holding, singing, talking, kissing and cuddling their firstborn son.

"I am grateful that I was so sick because we got three days with him. He did not leave our side and he slept in a baby crib right beside me for three whole nights. The midwives even kissed him goodnight and tucked him in."

Every moment together was precious, and Melinda expressed how lucky they felt being able to have that time because it is all they will ever have with him.

By the third day, Melinda and Lincoln noticed how rapidly Declan's delicate skin had changed. His skin had become so fragile that it was coming off his hand, making them hesitant to touch him too much in case they caused more damage.

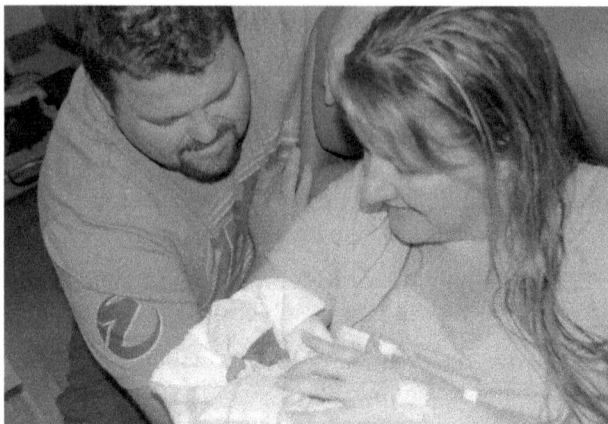

Melinda and Lincoln holding Declan

Leaving Declan was the worst part of Melinda's hospital experience. She was given a Bears of Hope bear so she would not leave the hospital empty-handed and this was an appreciated kindness at a time of great darkness.

"The pain of leaving Declan was excruciating. I really thought the emotional pain was actually going to kill me. I had to be physically pulled through the hospital doors, screaming because I wanted to stay with my baby. It's a day I will never forget, the absolute hardest thing I have ever had to do."

To this day, if Melinda has to visit that hospital, she does not use those doors. She will go out of her way to use another entrance because of the memories it evokes.

The couple drove home in silence. Married for less than a year, their hopes and dreams were shattered. Instead of celebrating the beautiful addition to their family, they had to arrange a funeral.

Declan's service took place two weeks later because Melinda just could not deal with it immediately. With help from Lincoln and her parents, she managed to go and look for the right place to bury him. It had to be somewhere she felt happy to visit, with a tree to provide shade. Melinda hates the heat and had always wanted to be buried under a tree, so she figured Declan needed the same. They eventually found the perfect place in Macquarie Park, amongst other babies and under a leafy tree.

Melinda wanted to see Declan one more time before the funeral.

"They decompose and change very quickly so they said no. I was angry at the world because they wouldn't let me see him. I was just so angry."

Following a beautiful service at a local Catholic Church, they took Declan to be buried and then had a wake at the home of Melinda's parents.

"The thing I wasn't prepared for was that a baby in a shoebox coffin still goes down six feet. I wasn't ready for that. You turn up at the cemetery and there's a massive gaping hole."

The couple visited Declan's grave often in the first few months. It was the only thing that got Melinda out of the house. She spent hours on the couch, staring at the wall. It only took the smallest thing to trigger a flood of tears. Adding to her pain was the medical information on the cause of Declan's death. Melinda's high blood pressure during pregnancy pumped her blood past the placenta rather than into it.

"I beat myself up. I was a mother and I failed my baby because he basically starved to death and I was unwell. I felt like it was my fault that he died and for many years I beat myself up. I didn't care if I died because my baby died, so I can too."

For months, Melinda physically sat still on the couch, while her mind and emotions ran rampant. Her memories are of a tough, dark and heavy time when her grief was inconsolable and sometimes very raw and ugly.

"In the early days, I threw a dog food can at the door and it exploded. I threw the TV remote at the mirror and broke the remote because that made me feel good for five seconds. For a few seconds I felt good, I got some of my anger out, and then I had a hell of a mess to deal with."

Melinda is not sure if it was a good or bad thing that Lincoln was also at home during these months. He spent most of his time on the computer searching for a new job while Melinda sat on the couch.

"I was really angry with the world. I was angry with myself. I was angry with everyone who got pregnant. I was angry with everyone who invited me to a baby shower. I was angry with everyone who had a healthy baby. They have one, why can't I? And I was angry at Lincoln because he didn't fix it."

Melinda recalls that in her distraught state, she couldn't understand why Lincoln wasn't sitting on the couch with her, crying his eyes out too. Now, she realises that men grieve differently and that they are often taught to hide their emotions. In contrast to Melinda, Lincoln internalised his grief and instead focussed on what he could do—find a job and provide for his family.

Life continued to move forward. Lincoln found work and Melinda gradually came back to life. At first, just getting up and having a shower was a triumph. It was one small step at a time.

I asked Melinda how she came from that terrible place to where she is today. A key factor for her was finding the right counsellor. Lincoln went to sessions with her initially then stopped, whereas Melinda continued on and still sees that counsellor five years on.

For Melinda, having the same counsellor throughout her journey has been incredibly beneficial in terms of not having to explain her history. The counsellor is able to continue on and can then deal with any new issues that arise.

> **"She made me feel normal. Because grief is extremely ugly. We do and say ugly things. She makes me feel like I'm not as bad or as ugly a person as I think I am."**

Lincoln and Melinda also sought to connect with other parents who had gone through a similar experience. They found a group and made new friends and it gave Lincoln a chance to speak and relate to other men dealing with the same kind of loss.

The support of Melinda's parents and siblings was unwavering, though some friendships have fallen by the wayside.

> **"We lost a lot of friends because people didn't know what to say to us, we were apparently too hard for them to deal with and made them too sad. That was a comment from a long-term friend. 'You make me too sad.' And I thought, 'Sorry for doing that to you for two minutes – try living through this hell!'"**

Around six months later, Melinda was scrolling through Facebook and noticed a charity that made angel gowns. It was a new not for profit organisation that provided bereaved families with angel gown packages free of charge. The concept was simple: they invited donations of wedding dresses which would be repurposed into many angel gowns by volunteer seamstresses. These would be offered to hospitals, providing both dignity and respect to the baby and the grieving family.

Melinda thought back to the clothes provided for Declan and remembered that all the hospital had available was a dolls outfit. She was intrigued.

> **"I thought this could be a way to channel my grief into something good, so I enquired. They asked if I could sew. I said no. Could I knit? Again, I had to say no. Crotchet? That was a no too. Then they asked if I was a good organiser and I said yes, yes, yes!!! And just like that I became area manager for Sydney."**

From that moment, Melinda found her purpose. Before long, her home was filled with wedding dresses and packages. Her mother became involved as well, sewing keepsakes to match the gowns, and making hearts used for silent funerals—the baby funerals no one attends. Melinda was quickly promoted to NSW Manager and coordinated seamstresses and volunteers who would knit and crochet blankets, booties and beanies. She also arranged the distribution of packages to hospitals and funeral homes.

Melinda returned to teaching and continued to coordinate the angel gown project on the side. She joined the charity's board and for three years, she devoted every spare moment to the organisation.

> **"I would deal with grieving families on my doorstep and send out urgent packages as needed. I was suddenly using my grief in a more positive way, helping others in their darkness, but mothering my own child at the same time. I have comforted strangers and later even befriended ladies crying at the cemetery. We are all connected through our grief."**

During these busy years, Melinda was more determined than ever to have a baby. Over the space of two and a half years, she had seven losses. Some were chemical pregnancies*, another was non-viable due to a chromosomal abnormality, another two were blighted ovums*. One baby was 10 weeks old and another, 8 weeks old. It was frustrating, heartbreaking and soul destroying.

> **"Declan changed my thinking forever. Peeing on a stick, finding out I was pregnant, there was no excitement anymore. I would just think, 'Here we go again,' because now I knew that nothing is certain."**

The stages of pregnancy became checkpoints: two lines on a stick, tick; blood test confirmed, tick, hCG doubling, tick, heartbeat tick. Getting past each step gave her a little relief because failure meant no baby.

In 2016, Melinda turned 39. Aware that the prime years for conception were slipping away, Melinda's mum suggested a change and asked her daughter to think about taking a year off teaching. At first, Melinda thought that going without a year's income was a crazy idea, but after serious consideration, she realised that it was possible. This led to her decision to move to different school in a casual teaching role.

At around the same time, Melinda heard a radio ad about Genea ovulation tracking. This involved a simple blood test to determine ovulation and the best time for conception. The couple had not had problems conceiving, but Melinda felt that she needed to change what she was doing to get a pregnancy to hold.

Melinda laughed as she described the moment when she found out the results—they were heading to a Swans football game on the train when she received the call saying that they needed to 'do it' by midnight that night and again before 7am the next morning! She hung up the phone and relayed the message to Lincoln. "But we're going to a Swans game!" he exclaimed. "You'll work it out!" she told him.

Melinda made sure that they got the job done and within two weeks they found out she was pregnant. Again, she felt terrified of going through all the stress and disappointment, but these emotions were over-ridden with her desperation to have a baby in her arms.

Due to her history, Melinda was cared for by an obstetrician who specialised in high-risk pregnancies. His calm manner was reassuring to the anxious couple. At their first scan, they saw two babies in separate sacs —twins!

Two weeks later, they returned to see only one heartbeat.

> **"Each time I went in for a scan I was stressed. Stressed out of my mind. Waiting for those words, 'There's no heartbeat, shut off the machine.' I was waiting for something bad to happen. I would go in, white as a ghost and the doctor would say, 'Can I do your blood pressure?' I would say, 'No, can we please see the heartbeat first?' So, he would show me the baby's heartbeat and once I saw it, I could relax. That's how I was for the whole pregnancy."**

By 20 weeks, Melinda was having weekly scans and as each week passed, it was a little easier emotionally. The pregnancy progressed normally, and three days before the due date, Melinda was admitted for induction.

After a brief scare when the medical staff were unable to find a heartbeat, Melinda asked to keep the monitor on her stomach throughout the night.

Watching the baby's heartbeat on the machine while she waited made her feel some degree of control because she could see that all was well.

At 4am, a nurse came in and ordered her to go to sleep, saying that she needed rest before going into labour in the morning. Melinda replied, "After my history, I need to watch this machine. I can rest tomorrow."

The nurse left and Melinda bawled. She was so upset at the way the nurse had spoken to her, feeling totally misunderstood and judged. Fortunately, a kinder midwife came in later and reassured her that the monitor would be watched from the nurse's station so she could sleep peacefully.

Melinda's doctor had administered gel overnight to get labour started but by morning, nothing had happened. He decided to reapply the gel and advised that the baby was likely to arrive before midnight and that they should go for a coffee to get the ball rolling. The predicted timing turned out to be a gross overestimate. At the hospital's coffee shop, Melinda started to have intense contractions, so they returned immediately to the birthing suite. Within two hours, Hudson was born.

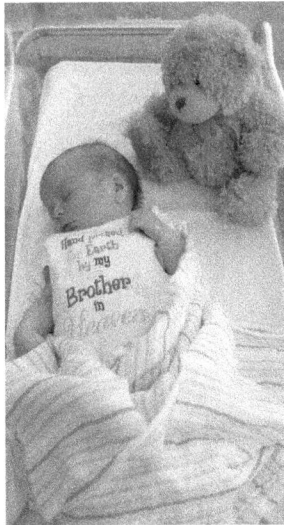

Hudson with Declan's Bear

"I was so relieved. There was a storm happening outside, and a rainbow came out. And he's my rainbow baby. And I'm thinking, this is all so perfect. Here he is, and he's mine and I just wouldn't let him go. He was my baby and he was here. Nothing else really mattered, they were stitching me up and it

really hurt, but it didn't matter. I didn't care. This was my baby. And I still haven't let him go. I have only gone back to work one day a week, so I spend my time mothering Hudson in real life, and mothering Declan through my charity work."

Melinda continues to raise Hudson, a very bright and delightful toddler. Her charity work has increased with the end of her relationship with the angel gown charity through controversial and hurtful circumstances. With one of the seamstresses, the two women decided that they could create their own charity.

"We came up with the name 'Made with Love—Murrum'. Murrum is an Aboriginal word that means beautiful, as the lady I am working with is Aboriginal."

Made with Love—Murrum works on a pledge system where people can promise their wedding dresses and once the dress is no longer needed, the donor sends it directly to the seamstress. This saves Melinda's home from being taken over with wedding gowns. She then co-ordinates all the other bits and pieces and makes up the packs that include gowns for girls and rompers for boys to make it easy to dress the fragile babies; blankets, keepsakes, beanies, cards, nappies, booties and more.

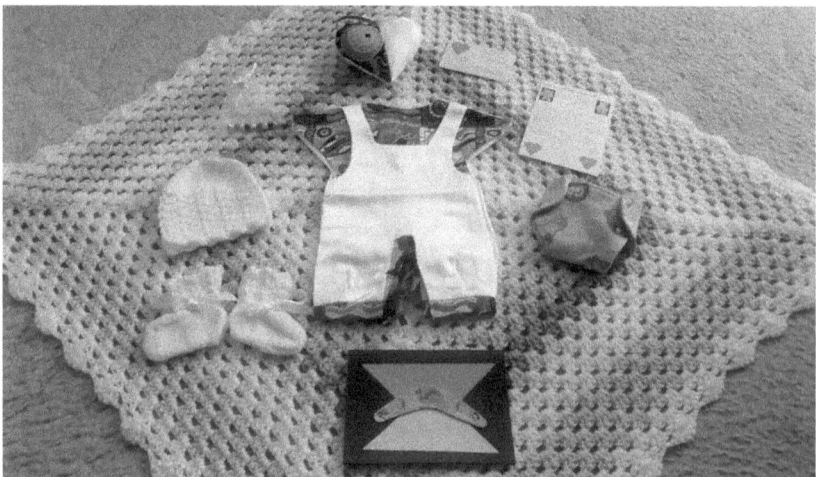

One of the beautiful Made with Love—Murrum packs

The packs are sized for age, from 10 weeks to 40 weeks and every pack is different, individually handmade with love. They have even created packs to cater for specific needs respecting the Aboriginal and Asian cultures.

Melinda's work has received well-deserved awards including the "Rising Star Award" from Women with Altitude. Her other ongoing charity work, tagging bears for Bears of Hope, has also been recognised with an award for "Volunteer of the Year" in 2018.

Following Hudson's birth, Melinda turned 40 and they knew that they had to move fast if they wanted to add more children to their family. After two more early miscarriages, the couple decided to try IVF.

"We tried a cycle of IUI and then IVF. We had one embryo put back in, but it didn't take. There's only so much science can do. Nature has to take over. We then changed companies and found a very caring and positive doctor and have since had two more cycles with a similar outcome – an embryo transferred for each cycle but not implanting itself in the final step."

Whether or not they add to their family, Melinda continues her important work honouring Declan by helping to provide a 'tiny touch of comfort' to other grieving families.

Lincoln and Melinda also include Hudson on their visits to the cemetery. Each year on Declan's birthday, they celebrate by going to the cemetery early and then going on to do a family activity that would have been age appropriate for that birthday. They finish the day with a butterfly or balloon release and seafood platter by the same lagoon each year. This year they went to Symbio Wildlife Park and Melinda did the Lemur experience for Declan.

"One of the hardest things about having a child in heaven and a child here on earth is having people say, 'Oh this your first— how wonderful.' I always correct them and say he has a brother in Heaven because my mother's guilt kicks in and I need to acknowledge both sons or I give myself grief for being weak and not sticking up for Declan.

This is hard to understand for those who haven't been where I am, but I know I need to do what is right for my own conscience."

Every day, Melinda looks for butterflies, her way of connecting with Declan in her daily life. She sees then in the park, at the beach, at the train station—everywhere. She believes that Declan comes to her in the form of butterflies and it warms her heart when they appear. Hudson has even learnt to point out butterflies to his mummy.

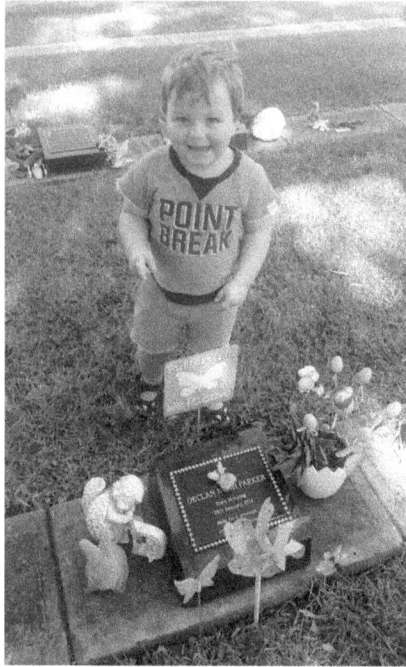

Hudson on a visit to Declan's grave

"You don't have to justify yourself to anyone else. That's a really important thing. We worry about what society is going to think, who cares? It's you and it's your world. I'm living this, and I'm doing it my way."

5

KATHERINE

- Ava, aged eleven, Epilepsy*
- Charlotte, aged seven
- Pre-eclampsia
- Gestational Diabetes
- Uterine Atony*
- Four Miscarriages
- Rainbow baby: Archer, aged six months

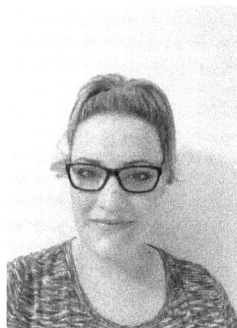

K atherine is one of those level-headed people that you wish for in a crisis situation. This might have something to do with her career, which started in nursing, and then continued in various capacities within sales for the healthcare industry. But I think it speaks more to the capable person she is in her roles as daughter, mother and wife.

Her first pregnancy was not planned. Katherine and her husband Glen conceived their first child when she was aged 30. The pregnancy progressed until the latter part of the third trimester when Katherine developed pre-eclampsia. This condition can be life-threatening to mother and baby, so her doctor recommended inducing the baby at 37 weeks.

Ava came into the world via forceps* delivery. A healthy girl, she grew up without any medical issues until the age of eight. One night, Katherine had arranged for Ava to stay with her parents because she was flying to Adelaide for work the next morning on a 6.30am flight. At about 3.30am, Katherine's father called saying, 'Ava's had a fit."

> **"I asked, 'What do you mean she's had a fit? Is she breathing?'
> Dad said, 'She's not responsive.' He was obviously panicking. I
> said, 'But is she breathing?' And he said, 'Yes.' I went straight
> over."**

By the time Katherine arrived, Ava was completely out of it. Katherine
checked her temperature and it was fine. From her nursing background,
she knew that once the seizure episode is finished, there's nothing you can
do. There is no test that can be done to see if you had a seizure or not.

Despite Katherine's assurances, her parents were 'freaking out'. She asked
them to take Ava to the doctor later that day, saying that she was only on a
day trip and would be back later that afternoon.

As expected, the doctor could not do anything, but he did refer Ava to the
Children's Hospital. Katherine's parents took her there. When Katherine
returned, the neurologist booked Ava in for a sleep test, but the
appointment was six weeks away. He suggested that they start Ava on
medication immediately.

Katherine knew that the medication could interfere with the sleep test
results, so she thought it better to delay starting anything until they had a
conclusive diagnosis.

> **"He said, 'Well, there's a 90% chance she'll probably have
> another seizure.' I said, 'For six weeks, I'll just take my
> chances.' And sure enough, she has another seizure. They
> thought, 'This mother is a nut.' But she didn't have asthma or
> anaphylaxis* or something, but with epilepsy, if you're in a
> safe position during the seizure you'll come out of it."**

After six weeks, Ava started on the medication and the sleep test revealed
brain activity that confirmed a diagnosis of epilepsy. Katherine tells me
that there have been some studies done linking forceps delivery with
epilepsy, and she wonders if that is what affected Ava.

The Epilepsy Foundation came out to the family and school and trained
everyone on how to administer Ava's medication. She was prescribed
Midazolam*, a drug used before surgery that they have found to be useful
in stopping seizures.

As Katherine described a few of Ava's episodes, I could see that she was
the one in the family who always keeps a cool head while everyone else
falls apart. One time, they were again at her parents' house and Ava had a
seizure. Katherine asked her mum to call the ambulance while she took
care of the medication. Her dad was crying, her mum couldn't speak to

the ambulance, and I visualised the scene that Katherine described: grabbing the phone from her mother, holding it in the crook of her neck and talking to the ambulance, holding Ava's head as she was vomiting, and trying to keep her daughter still so that she could give her the injection.

I asked Katherine how she stayed so calm during these episodes.

> **"I think I just felt that she was safe. Even though epilepsy can be threatening, I didn't feel that flight or fight, the feeling of being in an emergency. And the ambulances come really quick."**

When Ava was four, Glen and Katherine had Charlotte, now aged seven. From about 16 weeks into her second pregnancy, Katherine had gestational diabetes. This meant learning about the effects of certain foods, and also injecting insulin three times a day.

> **"It was a pain because you have to check your sugar two hours after you eat and the parameters for being pregnant are lower than when you are normal. I think my sugar had to be under 7.1, and you know how hard it is when someone says you can't eat now for two hours, because then all I'm doing is thinking about food."**

Charlotte was born at 39 weeks and five days via vacuum assisted delivery*. Katherine recovered well and at her six-week glucose tolerance test, her gestational diabetes was gone.

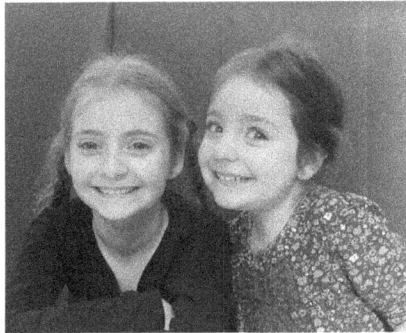

Ava and Charlotte

A few years later, the couple decided to add to their family. Katherine had no trouble falling pregnant. Their first scan showed a heartbeat and because of their two previous pregnancies, they fully expected this one to follow the same sequence.

At 10 weeks, the gestational diabetes had come back, and Katherine was attending her antenatal appointments as well as consulting an endocrinologist. She started spotting and checked with her doctor to see if that was normal.

> **"They said there can be spotting. I didn't really know about miscarriages. I just thought if you miscarried, everything starts bleeding and it all happens now. And I thought, well if they're not worried about it, then this must not be a big deal."**

The bleeding became worse and Katherine decided to go to the hospital. It was a Friday night and the doctor did a blood test. Once he had the results, he told her she was still very much pregnant.

> **"Of course, it would show as pregnant because your hormones don't just drop off. I said, 'But you haven't done anything. You haven't checked the heartbeat.' He was very dismissive."**

Katherine went home and said to Glen, "Something's not right." She went back to the hospital the next day on her own and had an ultrasound. The sonographer turned the screen and said, "I'll show you what I'm looking at. There's a foetus but there's no heartbeat." Then she cleaned up the gel and told Katherine that an orderly would come and get her.

The news that her baby had died was delivered without a shred of empathy. Worse still, Katherine was then wheeled into what appeared to be a closed ward in an isolated part of the hospital. She waited for over an hour, on her own.

When the doctor finally arrived, he confirmed the miscarriage, and said, "You can let it go naturally. It will be just like a heavy period, and we can book you in to an early pregnancy clinic and they can decide whether you have a curette or go natural." And that was it.

Katherine had no idea what to expect. She went home, just as her husband and mother were heading out to the Melbourne Salami Festa. They had both worked hard to make a salami sausage for this annual event, so Katherine told them to go ahead without her. The girls were already at Katherine's sister's place, so it gave her a little time to herself to think. She decided to get in the car and go for a drive to clear her head.

Different scenarios played out in her mind. The last thing she wanted to do was to wait for a week for something to happen. Katherine had been driving around for about 20 minutes, when she felt something wet and looked down to see the creases of her black pants pooling with blood. She was wearing a blue hoodie and the blood was creeping up, turning it red.

"I rang my husband and said, 'I'm going back to hospital because I'm bleeding a lot more now, it's pooling.' And he said, 'Pull over and call an ambulance.' I said, 'Don't be ridiculous. I'm not going to call an ambulance because I got a heavy period, don't be stupid.'"

She reached an intersection where, if she turned left, it would lead directly to the hospital. If she went straight, it would take her home.

"I suppose my way of coping with it was to become quite practical. I thought, 'I can go home, and I'll change my hoodie and my pants.' Because I was going to park in the shopping centre next door because it's free. I didn't want to park at the hospital because I'd have to pay a fortune. But if I parked at the shopping centre, I'd have to walk, but I didn't want to walk in these clothes because you could see all the blood."

Then she realised that she probably didn't have time to get home and reluctantly drove straight to the hospital and parked in their carpark. The bleeding was so excessive that there was no chance of cleaning off the blood—they had to replace the whole car seat!

Walking awkwardly through the carpark in her thongs, Katherine remembered something that a friend had told her. That friend was the only person she knew who had miscarried, and she remembered her describing it as feeling like an egg was coming out. As Katherine schlepped her way to the emergency department, she experienced that exact feeling.

By the time Katherine arrived at triage, the blood had run down her legs and reached her thongs. She was leaving a red trail on the ground behind her.

"There was a queue and I've just gone straight to the window. I said, 'I'm bleeding all over the floor.' She held up a pad and I said, 'I'm beyond that pad, love.'"

The nurse took her straight through and placed a pad on the bed. Within seconds, it was bright red, as if someone had poured cordial all over it. The medical staff mobilised and prepped her for theatre.

At that moment Glen arrived. Being ever practical, Katherine remembered she had left her phone in the car and sent Glen to fetch it before someone stole it. By the time he got back, Katherine had been transferred to a wheelchair and the blood loss had caused her to pass out.

When Katherine woke up, she had been fitted with an oxygen mask in the resuscitation bay. She was bleeding profusely and was told that she was going straight to theatre or she would bleed out.

"I was relieved because finally something was happening, there was an end to it and so then I could deal with it. I went to theatre and I felt so much better."

After surgery, Katherine was taken to a ward where Glen, her parents, her sister and brother-in-law came to visit. Her own clothes were ruined, so her sister went off to buy some new ones. Katherine felt so much better that she was able to sit up and eat ice-cream. A short time later, she needed to go to the bathroom and because she was still dressed in her gown, all open at the back, her parents and brother-in-law left the room to give her some privacy.

Katherine came back to the bed and sat on the edge, feeling awful. Glen asked her to move further back onto the bed and just as she shifted, her sister arrived back from shopping and Katherine collapsed.

"My sister thought I was dead, because my hands were contorted, I was grey, like a body. The nurse hit the emergency button and issued a MET* call. So, my parents are outside and there are so many people rushing in. My sister comes out and she thinks I'm dead. They sent them into a family room. My mum was taken to a family room when her dad died, so they're all thinking I'm dead, and really I've just passed out from blood loss."

Katherine woke up, fitted with the oxygen mask again and a group of people staring at her from the end of her bed. She was banned from getting up for any reason and ordered to stay overnight.

The hospital had arranged for Katherine to see her GP for her postpartum check-up. At that stage, they had no information on the cause of the miscarriage or if it was safe to try again. He blithely advised her, "Get over it. It was a miscarriage, just let it go, don't worry about it."

"That made me angry. I stopped going to see him after that. There was no support. I didn't know what my options were. No

one from the hospital contacted me. It was like it didn't matter. I was treated like I didn't have any right to feel it was valid."

Usually, testing is not arranged until after three miscarriages. Because of the dramatic impact of Katherine's miscarriage, testing was conducted, even though this was her first. Her new GP delivered the results, explaining that her baby had Trisomy 15*, an extremely rare chromosomal disorder.

"What did that mean? How could that have happened? They look at me and think that because I've had two kids, it was just random bad luck."

Katherine could not believe the lack of information provided. She expected to get an explanation of why it happened. And if the GP didn't know, then surely, he would arrange testing on herself and Glen, or at least refer them to a genetics specialist.

None of this was offered, and the couple fell pregnant six months later. Katherine noticed that she was more apprehensive, now fully aware that pregnancy does not always result in a healthy baby.

At the first scan, baby measured well with a healthy heartbeat. By the next ultrasound, the heartbeat had gone. Katherine was booked in for D & C but had to wait to be fitted in.

"There was no sense of urgency when you've had a loss. There's no recognition that some people don't want to go through the natural process. People like me don't want to wait. If you tell me right now it's finished, then I want to have a curette, just take me straight to theatre. But there's no sense of urgency, because it's not a medical emergency. There's no consideration of your mental well-being in between that time of finding out, to when you have a curette."

At this point, Katherine and Glen consulted a gynaecologist. He arranged for them both to be tested, thinking that they might have an imbalance in their chromosomes. The results showed that neither of them had any issues. He suggested that the cause might simply be age and he encouraged them to keep trying.

Katherine's fifth pregnancy followed the same pattern. At around 10 weeks, she was in Sydney on a work trip when the spotting began. As soon as her plane touched down in Melbourne, Katherine contacted her GP who arranged an appointment with the gynaecologist in hospital the following day.

By the time she arrived at the hospital, the bleeding had increased, so Katherine was taken immediately to theatre for a D & C. The surgeon explained that the extreme blood loss was due to Uterine Atony, a serious condition where the uterus fails to contract.

The gynaecologist sent the tissue away for testing while Katherine recovered. That baby would have been born with Turners Syndrome* a chromosomal abnormality that only affects girls. Again, with Katherine now 40, the doctors suggested it was likely because of her age.

By this time, the couple had become familiar with the process and Katherine decided that she wanted her tested tissue sample returned.

> **"I emailed and thought, 'They'll think I'm weird because I want my stuff,' but there was no issue and they accommodated that quite well and so that side was good. Some people may not want it back but at least it should be an option that you can request it, because they wouldn't know. I got it back and put it inside a Build-A-Bear, and that did give me some closure. Like it did matter."**

Katherine and Glen decided to try one more time and after easily falling pregnant again, that pregnancy followed the same pattern and resulted in their fourth miscarriage.

The effect of the miscarriages has rippled out to the whole family. When the first miscarriage occurred, Ava was at an age where she wanted to know why it had happened. Katherine and Glen explained that we are made up of DNA and chromosomes and that the baby had three of a particular type of chromosome that meant that it couldn't survive.

Recently, when chatting with Ava about the future, growing up and having children, Katherine realised that the miscarriages have had a big impact on everyone in the family.

> **"Ava said, 'Oh, I don't know if I'll have any kids.' I said, 'Why do you think you won't have kids?' And she said, 'I might have a miscarriage.'"**

Katherine's experiences have obviously shaped Ava's thinking, but Katherine also feels that part of the problem is that people don't talk about it.

"It's not until you talk about it, until you've been through it and you talk to other people that they say, 'Oh, I had one.' People around you are very uncomfortable, they don't know what to say. They sometimes say quite hurtful things that make you feel like you have no reason to grieve, that it's not a valid person. They say very unhelpful things like, 'Oh, you've got two, you should be grateful for those two.' But if you had three children and one died, no one would say that."

I asked Katherine how she moved forward from those places of grief. As a pragmatic and practical person, she needed to know why things had happened. She's the type of person who realises that they can't go back and change the past. She felt that time, information and understanding about what had happened helped her to deal with her emotions.

"I think having them tested and finding out the sex helped. The first and third were girls and that gives them an identity. In some ways that made it a bit harder, because then you can picture what you've lost. But I think having answers and the medical reasons helped me to deal it."

One of the most difficult things to handle was the triggers. Katherine would see pregnant women everywhere she went. When it was past her due date, she would see a newborn and could not help but think that her child would have been at that same stage. Seeing or having anything to do with children who would have been the same age was difficult.

"Every now and again, I don't think you ever forget, it still comes back up."

Katherine's treatment by the healthcare professionals did not help. She feels that the industry as a whole should remember that we are whole people, and not just a physical body.

"I didn't realise just how clinical they are. After my first ultrasound, I had retained products of conception. I understand where they are coming from, but it's very clinical and very much treating the physical side of it, not at all taking into account your mental state."

After their fourth, they agreed that they could not keep going through the process again and again.

"Clearly my eggs weren't fine two years ago, and they're not going to be better quality now. So, let's just stop. And also because of the history of bleeding. I didn't want to leave that cloud hanging over us. So, we refitted out the last bedroom into a kid's area and study nook."

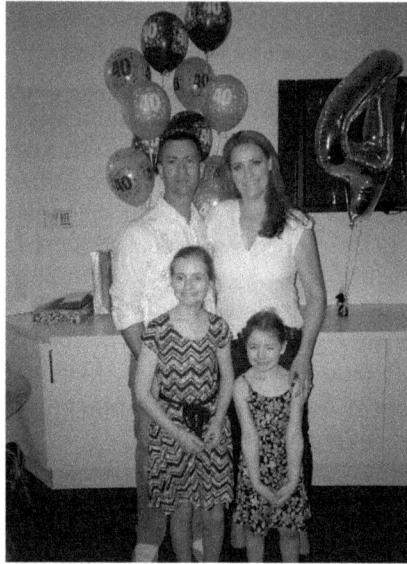

Glen, Katherine, Ava and Charlotte

Happy with their decision and the new home renovation, the family settled into the thinking that their family was complete. But in early 2019, Katherine was feeling a little bloated. She thought that she might be menopausal—her mother had started early—or maybe it was ovarian cancer!

There was no point worrying until she had a definitive diagnosis on what was causing the problem. Her doctor thought it might be a gynaecological issue and sent Katherine off for an ultrasound.

"Ever since I've had the miscarriages, I can't look at the screen. I hate walking in, even if I'm going for a hip ultrasound. The sonographer's looking at the screen and he's looking at me, like he wants to say something. And I think, oh, I'm dying, I've got tumours. And it turned out that I was 12 weeks pregnant."

Katherine was in absolute shock. She wrestled with dichotomous thoughts in her mind, ranging from, "Oh no, here we go again, I'm going to have to go through this all over again," through to "I'm so excited." It took a day to process her own emotions before she was able to tell Glen and her family.

> **"The first thing my daughter said when we told her that I was pregnant this time was, 'I hope you don't have another miscarriage.' They are so innocent, they just say what they think, so honest."**

Because they were already at 12 week's gestation, tests were organised straight away. Within days they had the Nuchal Translucency scan and blood screening test that takes into account the mothers age. At 41, Katherine was deemed to be of 'advanced maternal age' and the results suggested a high risk of Down Syndrome. A more in-depth and accurate test called a non-invasive prenatal test (NIPT)* was arranged, and those results came back as low risk of Down Syndrome.

These confusing results offered no reassurances. Every other indication showed a healthy pregnancy progressing well, but obviously the test results and previous experiences played on Katherine's mind.

> **"We found out that we're having a boy, which is what my husband had always wanted. But all the miscarriages have taken away the joy. As much as you want to be thrilled, it's always in the back of your mind that it might happen again."**

To give herself some peace of mind, Katherine purchased her own doppler* so that she could monitor the baby's heartbeat at any time. The next 16 weeks progressed well, then at 28 weeks, Katherine was diagnosed with gestational diabetes.

From this point forward, she needed to inject four doses of insulin per day. The baby was deemed Large for Gestational Age (LGA)* and required regular growth scans. By 36 weeks, he was in the 90th percentile for size!

When diabetes and advanced maternal age are factors in a pregnancy, induction at 38 weeks is recommended. The date was booked for 38 weeks and three days. Katherine went in as scheduled and began induction at 7.30am. It was a slow delivery, and at one point the baby's heart rate dropped. If the situation continued, a c-section would have to be performed.

Thankfully, the baby moved down far enough so that the doctor could deliver him with forceps. Archer was welcomed into the world at 6.43pm, 51cm long and weighing 3.59kg.

Mother and baby were so healthy that they were both discharged the next day. At the time of writing, Archer is just a week old and his parents are thrilled with their new son, bracing with trepidation for the upcoming sleepless nights!

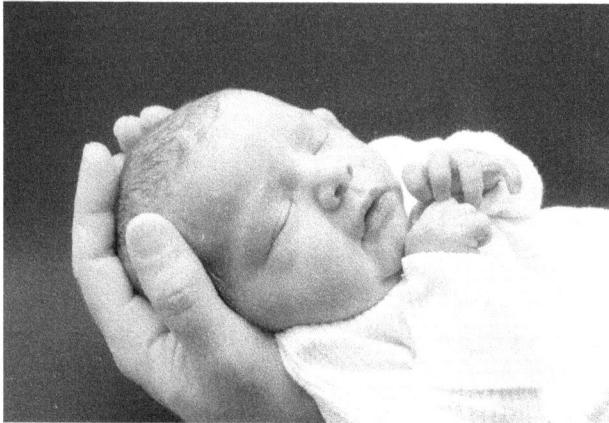

Archer

"Just because I was okay then, doesn't mean that in two weeks' time, when it all hits home, and I get my first period (because it's a trigger that reminds you of when you started spotting) that I'll be okay then. They don't say, 'Look, these are the things that might happen. You might think you're okay, but in two or three weeks you should be feeling better than you are now, but in fact, you can feel worse. If you do, call this number or come back and talk to someone.'"

6

SAMANTHA

- Sunshine baby Georgie, aged seven
- Two Miscarriages
- Rainbow baby Johnny, aged three
- Postnatal Anxiety
- Recent Miscarriage

As a child growing up in the North of England, Sam grew up in a town where it was normal to be a teenage parent— school leavers would often marry their sweetheart and have children before the age of 25.

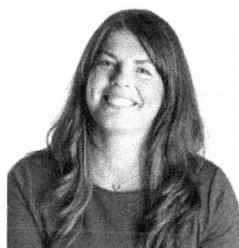

Sam met the man she would marry during university and they have been together since the age of 18. Instead of settling down, Sam and Stewart decided to explore the world, living and working in Portugal as a base. Then in 2009, they discovered Australia.

It was initially the traditional expat life of sun, sand and surf that attracted them to the country, but they soon realised that it would also be a wonderful place to raise a family. Upon making this decision, Sam fell pregnant with Georgie almost straight away.

> **"Georgie was the immaculate conception, easy pregnancy, bit of a rubbish labour, but that didn't really bother me, I was happy to have a c-section* and she was awesome. No problems whatsoever."**

Sam chose to take some time off from her teaching career to enjoy being a mum. She joined a local play group and it soon became obvious that she was one of the youngest mothers there.

"They kind of looked down at me, saying, 'Aren't you 30 yet?' I said, 'I'm 29, I'm not a child bride or anything.'"

It was probably just an innocent question, but to Sam, it was an example of how we judge people based on our own experiences and cultural norms. Compared to people in her hometown, Sam thought she had started her family much later than normal and here she was being questioned about her youth!

When Georgie was almost two years old, the couple decided to add to their family. Again, Sam fell pregnant almost immediately. Unsure of her conception date, she went in for a dating scan around what she thought was six weeks into her pregnancy.

The ultrasound showed a heartbeat, but she was told that the baby looked a little small. This information didn't mean anything to Sam. Her first pregnancy had gone as expected, without any complications, so she didn't even consider that there would be problem. The sonographer asked her to return in two weeks to confirm that everything was on track.

Over the following fortnight, a few questions crept into Sam's mind. She thought, "I didn't have to do that with Georgie, so why do I have to do that now?" Sam rationalised her worries and dismissed them with simple explanations such as, "Maybe the dates are wrong," to account for the baby's size. Besides, she still felt all of the usual signs of pregnancy.

With this in mind, Sam went to the check-up scan with only her toddler and without adult support. After a few movements of the ultrasound wand, the sonographer stopped abruptly and asked Sam to call her husband.

The worst possible scenarios instantly flooded through Sam's brain. She called Stewart immediately and it was fortunate that he was working close by.

Once he arrived, Stewart was ushered quickly into the treatment room. "I'm really sorry," said the sonographer. "There's no heartbeat."

"It's called a missed miscarriage," explained Sam. "That was really awful because even though there was a seed of doubt, we never expected that outcome. We genuinely thought that we would never lose the baby."

Sam praised the sonographer for delivering the news in a very empathetic way, appreciative of her care in providing them with the room for as long as they needed.

Stewart and Sam went home from the imaging centre, shattered and unsure of what they were supposed to do next. The sonographer informed Sam that she needed to see a GP to confirm the miscarriage. Georgie had been born through the public health system and the family didn't have a regular GP, so Stewart phoned the local medical centre to explain what had happened. They didn't have any free appointments but due to the circumstances, offered to fit Sam in to see a doctor.

The couple arrived at the medical centre, emotionally devastated. Stewart asked for a private room several times, but nothing was offered. They ended up sitting in the crowded reception area for over an hour.

Finally, they were called into one of the doctors' offices. The GP looked at the scans and was very matter-of-fact, saying, "This happens a lot. You'll be pregnant again before you know it. Don't worry about it. Here's the number for EPAS*." He scribbled on a yellow sticky note, handed it to them and showed them out.

> **"There was no empathy, no understanding. I've just been told the most devastating news ever, and he hands me a sticky note with a number. And I didn't even know what an EPAS clinic was. He didn't explain that there were different types of miscarriages, that I would potentially have to have surgery, there was nothing. I was literally in and out of his office in a couple of minutes."**

The doctor may have seen hundreds of miscarriage cases, but for Sam and Stewart, this was the first time their lives had been touched by miscarriage. The whole experience was new and traumatic. So many questions and emotions were crushing them, and they were not getting answers or appropriate care.

Hoping for some genuine support, Sam phoned the number on the note. She discovered that EPAS was the acronym for Early Pregnancy Assessment Service. The clinic was booked out and could not fit them in for three days.

> **"Those three days were torture. To know that your baby has passed away...for some women, they choose to miscarry naturally, and they'll wait with the baby inside of them. For me, I wanted closure. I wanted it to be done with. I didn't want to be pregnant anymore. I was angry at my body, so those few**

days were extremely difficult and totally screwed with my head. No other way to say it."

With no information provided by any health professional, Sam used Google to try and find out more about what had just happened to her and her baby. All she found were horror stories of individual women's journeys and this was not at all helpful. After extensive searches, Sam couldn't find any trusted sources of information or support.

"There wasn't anything that I needed available in terms of trying to explain what was happening to me, so I was in limbo."

Sam's visit at the EPAS Clinic gave her some much-needed facts. She explained to the nurse that she had not started bleeding and had waited for three days to get her appointment. The nurse was kind, explaining Sam's options with care and consideration. One choice she offered was a D & C procedure. This was the first time Sam had heard the term, and also the first indication that she might need to have surgery.

A theatre booking was available that morning and she was prepped immediately for surgery. Thinking back, Sam recalls how she went to that EPAS appointment completely unaware that an operation was a possibility —she was totally unprepared for it emotionally.

Adding to the psychological trauma was the fact that the procedure took place in the same hospital where Sam had given birth to Georgie two years prior. In fact, the recovery room she was taken to after the D & C was the exact same room where they placed Georgie in her arms after her c-section.

"Why would they do that? I get it, it's to do with procedures after surgeries, but it just didn't feel right and it made me angry."

The beautiful memories Sam had previously held about the hospital were now tainted with sadness and pain. She left feeling empty, confused and the sadness was overwhelming.

The worst part of Sam's experience was the lack of follow up. She sat at home with her grief, utterly alone, trying to make sense of the last two weeks—her excitement, expectation and joy of having a baby had been transformed into loss and self-blame.

At the time when she most needed support, there was nothing but blank silence from all the medical professionals she had encountered. No phone call to say, "Are you OK?" There were no referrals to support organisations, nor advice on when to try again.

There was also the matter of telling friends and family. As soon as she discovered she was pregnant, Sam had shared the news with everyone, saying how excited she was and how wonderful it would be to have two-and-a-half-years between Georgie and the baby.

Following the miscarriage, Sam had to deal with her own feelings while fielding questions from well-meaning loved ones. She decided to be open about it and found that some people were shocked that she was happy to talk about it.

"A few friends said, 'I've had one too.' I was like, 'Really? I had no idea! Why didn't you tell me?' They replied, 'Well you just don't talk about it.'"

Sam and I discussed this unspoken cultural understanding that miscarriage is not discussed. There's the common thinking that we shouldn't tell people about pregnancy until we are past the 12 week period, but this brings with it the issue that if we do not tell people about our pregnancy, and then experience an early loss, there is no validation that it happened at all. If we have not told you about being pregnant, then how can we tell you about our loss?

"Women feel that they shouldn't or that they are invalid in their grief. That's wrong, really wrong because it's not emotionally healthy. As Brené Brown advocates, if we share our stories, it removes the shame."

I asked Sam how she moved forward from that emotional state. Sam shared that she was a resilient person, and that she found that talking about her experience helped her to emerge from grief, to pick herself up and to get on with life. She did not put any pressure on herself to conceive immediately, instead choosing to enjoy the family she was so grateful to have.

Over the next few months, Sam processed her emotions of failure, reminding herself that she had already carried a healthy child. She had to change her feelings around the miscarriage from being her fault, to being a case of bad luck.

Just after the following New Year, Sam was shocked to find out that, unbeknownst to her, she had fallen pregnant sometime before Christmas. Anxiety and self-blame kicked in with thoughts that she'd had a few drinks over that period. If anything happened this baby, she would feel responsible, thinking that healthwise, she needed to be really 'clean' for a successful pregnancy.

> **"I was really worried this time. I felt like I'd been robbed, like I had my innocence taken away from me. That just because you're pregnant and you've got two lines on a test that doesn't mean you're going to have a baby at the end of it."**

There was a constant inner dialogue going in her head. One moment she reasoned that she'd had her bad luck and that this baby was going to be fine. Then the next moment, the fear of another miscarriage would take over.

In January, Sam went in for a dating scan, and everything was fine, but because she was nervous, the staff said to come back in a couple of weeks for another scan. That eight-week scan confirmed that the baby was measuring correctly and that there was a heartbeat—Sam was elated.

Shortly after that scan, the family went on an island holiday to Queensland with some friends. A few days in, Sam began to bleed, and her pregnancy symptoms faded. Her breasts were no longer sore, she wasn't feeling nauseous and she wasn't hungry all the time.

> **"I just knew. I had this deep-seated feeling. It wasn't fear, I knew I'd lost the baby. But I didn't tell anyone because I didn't want to ruin the end of what had been a really good week's holiday."**

I asked Sam why so many of us feel exactly the same way, putting other people's needs before our own.

> **"It's a woman thing. I felt silenced in my first miscarriage, but I felt even more silenced the second time around. When people didn't talk much about the first miscarriage, the subsequent time I internalised that previous experience as this being a subject that you don't speak about."**

Stewart knew something was wrong because of Sam's moodiness, but he had no idea what had happened until she told him on the night they returned home to Sydney. He still held out hope, but a scan the following morning confirmed the worst—there was no baby anymore.

Fortunately, there was an appointment available the following day at the EPAS Clinic. This time, however, she was warned that she may potentially miscarry at home overnight. Without further explanation or information provided, she was sent home.

That night, Sam woke up with contractions. She recognised them immediately from her past labour experience giving birth to Georgie. At 3am, Sam passed the baby alone in the shower.

"That was one of the lowest points for me."

And then she began bleeding profusely. Was it too much? There was nowhere else to turn except Google so she tried to get answers but again, could not find what she needed. Should she go to emergency? Sam had no idea. She didn't feel comfortable going to hospital, thinking,

"Would I be made a fool of? Will they just tell me that this is common, that I shouldn't be there and that I am wasting their time and should have stayed home?"

Sam arrived at the EPAS clinic at 7am that same morning.

"We both sat there, my husband and I, in a waiting room full of people who had probably gone through the same thing. No one was looking at each other, there was no eye contact. There was a sliver of hope in some people. You try not to cry because you don't want to upset other people."

When Sam's name was called, a female doctor ushered her into a treatment room. She noticed that the doctor appeared to be six or seven months pregnant. Sam immediately put herself in that doctor's place, thinking how awful it must be to work all day with women who had lost their babies.

"I felt guilty, and I said, 'I'm so sorry, this must be really difficult for you. You don't need to deal with me today.' In hindsight she should never have been working in that department."

It was actually quite a confronting situation, being treated by a woman whose body was doing exactly what Sam's had failed to do. Clearly no malice was intended, but if the scheduling staff had stopped to think about how a heavily pregnant woman would emotionally affect all of the EPAS Clinic patients, then perhaps they would have realised that it would have been better for her to work in a different department.

Scans showed that Sam had not passed all of the baby and that there was some tissue just outside of the uterus. The doctor performed a procedure there and then in the consulting room, literally putting her fingers inside, pulling out the tissue and putting it in a test tube.

The doctor placed the test tube in a petri dish on her desk and continued to talk to the couple. That was just too much—to Sam and Stewart, that was their baby, sitting on the doctor's desk right in front of them. They asked for it to be moved.

> **"To her, as the doctor, she probably sees 10 patients a day and it's become normalised for her. She's not insensitive, she's uneducated and unaware of the impact of her actions. It's the little things like that, that then traumatise women further down the line."**

Sam came home, absolutely bereft. She was a mess. The anxiety started to creep in with thoughts that she was never going to be able to have another child. One of the hardest things to cope with was the comments from people who would say, "At least you have Georgie."

These words may have been said with good intent, but for someone who has just lost their baby, it's a phrase that Sam firmly believes should never be said.

> **"Why is it at least? It's because Georgie is so amazing that I want another child. Why can't I have another child? There's no at least, because to me and to all of the women who go through this, that's your baby. It's as simple as that. From the moment you get those two lines, you imagine a future: whether it will be a boy or a girl, how you will decorate the nursery, what type of pram you'll have, what a wonderful big sister Georgie will be and what names you will choose. Your mind runs away with all that because it's such a time of joy and excitement."**

Sam realised that she needed support. She researched online and could only find charities who assisted families affected by stillbirth. At the time, Same felt that her grief was incomparable and that her personal situation did not warrant the help of those organisations.

Eventually, Sam found a Facebook group and saw an anonymous message that was filled with genuine compassion and empathy. Sam sensed that this person truly understood how she felt, so she reached out. That person turned out to be Gabbi, a woman who has endured years of IVF and has also experienced six miscarriages.

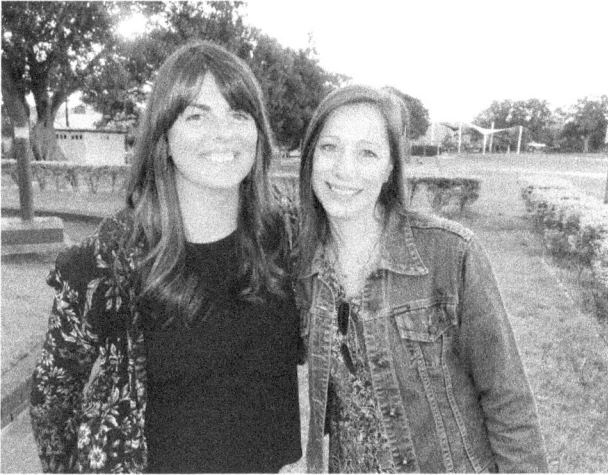

Sam and Gabbi

These two women decided to catch up for coffee and by the end of their conversation, the pair had agreed that there was a huge unmet need in the community around the support of women experiencing early miscarriage. The concept for Pink Elephants was born.

I asked Sam how they decided upon the name, and she told the beautiful story of how their research uncovered an old fable that gave them goosebumps—a sign that it was the perfect inspiration for their organisation. The story explains what happens when an elephant mother loses her baby. The other elephants form a circle of support around her and gently touch her with their trunks, allowing her all the time she needs to grieve and mourn.

> **"It's that silent unwavering show of support, that's all that's required when someone is going through miscarriage, and that's to actually be physically there for them."**

Sam and Gabbi set to work researching the best way to support women who, like them, had experienced early pregnancy trauma. They found a huge lack of support, not just in Australia but globally. In Australia there are currently 103,000 miscarriages a year and globally, 33 million. Statistically, that's one in four pregnancies ending in miscarriage, and one in three women experiencing miscarriage.

Pink Elephants supports women through their grief by providing access to relevant information about miscarriage. They provide beautiful, emotionally supportive resources and connections with other women. Sam and Gabbi have written the content from their lived experience of loss and all the resources have been reviewed and approved by leading obstetricians and gynaecologists.

Available on their website and distributed in early pregnancy clinics and hospital emergency departments, the resources have been exceptionally well received.

> **"We got amazing feedback. All the nurse unit managers were so grateful, saying, 'This is something that we're trying to help people with, but we haven't actually been through it. It's so nice that two women who have been through it are willing to share their journey and help others.'"**

The other important area that Sam and Gabbi wanted to address was peer support, helping women to connect with someone who had been through a similar experience. They established online support communities and their unparalleled Peer Support Program, provides six free phone sessions with a mentor who has lived experience of early pregnancy loss.

In March 2017, Pink Elephants achieved charity status and in 2019, Sam was crowned NSW winner of the Telstra Business Women's Award for Purpose & Social Enterprise.

> **"I was really proud to get the award. It was really incredible, an amazing experience to have what I've created being recognised and special, knowing that I have tangibly impacted thousands of women."**

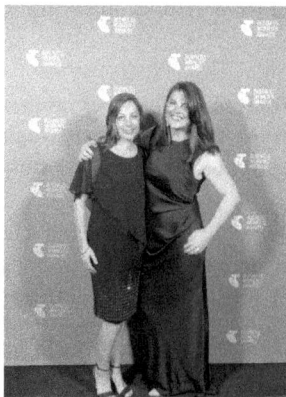

Gabbi and Sam at The Telstra Business Women's Awards

While striving to make a difference through Pink Elephants, Sam was facing her own health challenges. Following her second loss, Sam's body didn't feel right. She had a myriad of physical ailments including swollen joints, headaches and brain fog and an inability to lose her baby weight despite eating well. These are all symptoms associated with being a new mother.

Sam wanted to be in peak condition before conceiving again, so she went to see a gynaecologist. He told her that testing would only be done after a third miscarriage, and that if a baby has a genetic abnormality, if a baby is not meant to be, then she would miscarry. This was not enough of an explanation for Sam, it did not give her the confidence to try again.

Needless to say, Sam did not go back to that specialist, but instead, found a good naturopath through her GP. The naturopath suggested running some tests and Sam's GP arranged scans to check her uterus.

"I found out I had an MTHFR (methylenetetrahydrofolate reductase)* gene, a faulty gene that my husband tested for as well. It's called epigenetics*. Some medical professionals don't believe it has any effect, but all my physical symptoms were linked to it."

Sam began an intensive three-month health kick, giving up caffeine, sugar, dairy and processed food because they trigger the way that the gene is expressed. She also discovered that folic acid, an essential vitamin during pregnancy, was unsuitable for her in the synthetic supplement form. Her solution? To eat loads of fresh spinach and supplement with natural folate.

There's no way of telling whether or not this had any effect, but it gave Sam a much-needed feeling of power and control, something that was vitally important at the time. It gave her focus because they were real steps she could take to positively determine the outcome of her next pregnancy.

Four months later, Sam fell pregnant. The pregnancy was physically fine, but Sam was not coping mentally or emotionally. In hindsight, she realises that instead of burying her emotions, she should have sought counselling.

Adding to her trauma was Sam's continued work with Pink Elephants. Sam found that she was comparing herself to others, telling herself that she had no right to feel awful when so many women were in a worse situation that she was…Sam felt she should feel grateful to be pregnant.

"I was trying to detach, not to attach to this baby. I just didn't want to talk about being pregnant, and almost wanted to ignore that I was pregnant, so I didn't share that in the early stage because I thought, 'What's the point? It will probably end up in miscarriage anyway.'"

On top of this emotional turmoil, the family suffered more loss. In the UK, Stewart's nephew died suddenly in a car accident when Sam was six months pregnant.

"It was awful, I couldn't fly back for the funeral because I was a high-risk pregnancy. Then we lost my husband's dad a few weeks later."

Despite the geographical distance between them and their relatives, the family is extremely close. Not physically being there was incredibly difficult. The joy of Johnny's birth was tempered with the loss of loved ones. Adding to that, was the fact that he was a very sick newborn. When Johnny was just one week old, they suspected he had meningitis* and the doctors decided that they needed to perform a lumber puncture*.

"My husband couldn't be in the room. He said, 'I can't be here', and I thought, 'Well I can't leave him,' so I had to watch them pin him down as a baby. It was the worst."

Johnny did not have meningitis, but he did succumb to lots of colds and viruses. This resulted in him being in and out of hospital for the first few months of his life. Johnny cried constantly and was a restless and upset baby. Looking back, Sam believes that it was her anxiety being transferred over to him. When Johnny was around four months old, Sam was diagnosed with postpartum anxiety.

"I wasn't depressed, I didn't want to check out or have suicidal thoughts. I permanently worried that Johnny would die. I wouldn't put him down, I wouldn't let anyone else hold him, I just wanted to keep him away."

It was a few words from Gabbi, "You're not right. I'm worried about you," that finally made Sam seek help. She went to her GP and asked for a mental health assessment.

"We have this perception that if you need a mental health plan, you're crazy. Whereas it's actually a validation that you've been through a traumatic time that has induced this stress in your body and you now need this mental support to process it, let it go and move on. If you don't do all those things, you just fall in a heap."

The GP referred Sam to a psychologist and prescribed her with medication. Within two weeks, she was a different person.

"I needed that medication at that time, something to level me back to earth, to stop the constant train of worry going around my head. Because all these people died, I lost all these babies and I just felt everyone was going to die."

Sam moved forward gradually. The medication stopped the destructive thoughts enough to get some sleep, while the counselling helped her to articulate those thoughts and to identify the journey she had been on.

By talking with a professional, Sam could see that the timing of Pink Elephants had not been the best for her personally. It was too much. While she was dealing with the miscarriages and pregnancy with Johnny, she had been internalising everyone else's grief and not processing her own. Sam was constantly triggering herself every day but continued because she could see the greater good and the way her work was positively impacting people. But it wasn't healthy for her own wellbeing.

"As I got better, Johnny got better too. He is now one of the most chilled out kids. He's so totally different."

Sam recently fell pregnant again and understandably, she was nervous to be going through pregnancy after loss again. She described it as "never quite fully believing that you will have a baby in your arms."

Sharing her news with her #circleofsupport, Sam reached each milestone of increasing hCG levels, the first scan with a sac in the right place, another scan with a heartbeat and baby measuring correctly. She gradually let herself believe that this baby would soon be holding her third child.

However, a week after a scan with a strong heartbeat, Sam started to bleed. She instantly knew she had lost her baby. Sam's GP referred her to the EPAS who confirm the loss, just as they had before. She chose to have another D & C because the trauma of another natural miscarriage was not something she wanted to ever go through again.

"It feels cruel, pointless and really unfair that I am here again bearing this pain. I am however supported by my #circleofsupport. My loss has been validated with beautiful gestures of support that have been really cathartic. I feel that society is changing the narrative on early pregnancy loss and recognising the trauma and lasting impact."

Sam is really grateful that she had access to bereavement leave, something she never had with her last losses. This gave her the time and space to grieve and when the waves of grief felt too much to bear, she could sit at home and grieve. She didn't need to return to work and wear a mask pretending everything was normal or that she was okay.

Realising the need for other women to be afforded the same opportunity, Sam and the team at Pink Elephants are working with the University of Sydney to spearhead a campaign for legislative change around bereavement leave after miscarriage. You can find out more about he Leave for Loss campaign on the Pink Elephants website.

Today Sam continues to grow all aspects of Pink Elephants. The charity collaborates with the University of Melbourne to conduct research which can be translated into meaningful services. They offer education programs for medical professionals to make them aware of the impact of their words and actions on patients. Sam continues to fundraise so that Pink Elephants can continue to 'fill the gap' within the perinatal space for women.

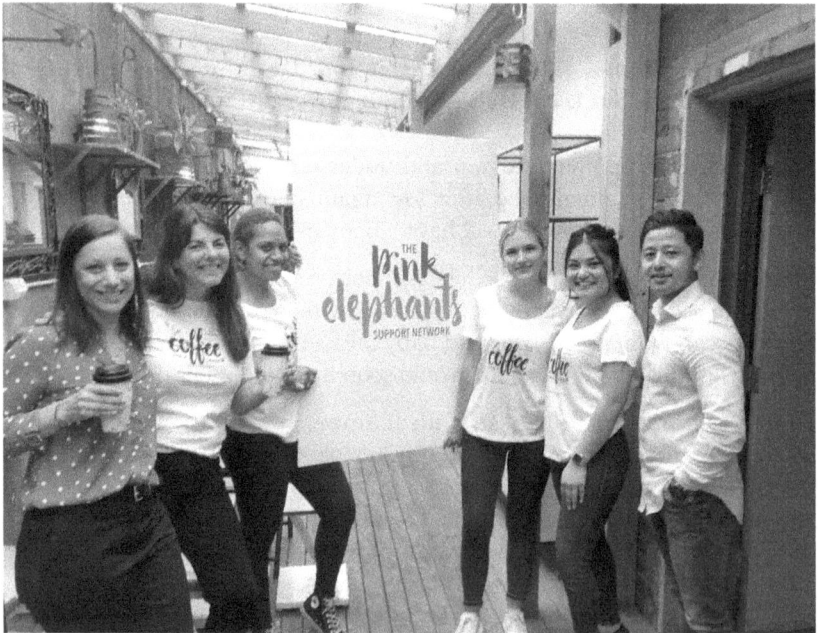

The Pink Elephants Team

"Connect with other women who have been there and can normalise that it is okay to feel really anxious one day, and really grateful the next day. Each day is very different. You also need someone to acknowledge for you that this is a different pregnancy, a different baby, and a different outcome. These three things are really important."

7

AMANDA

- Angel baby, Eva
- Gestational Diabetes
- Rainbow baby Lillian, aged three. Born with Low Blood Sugar and Jaundice
- Two Miscarriages
- New Pregnancy

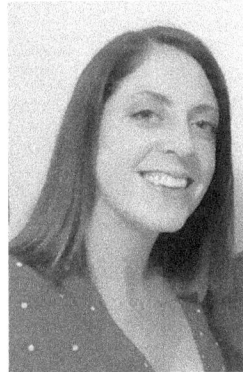

The youngest of four children, Amanda's conception was a happy 'accident'. By the time of her birth, her two sisters had grown up and left home, and only her 12-year old brother still lived at home.

Born five weeks premature, Amanda's traumatic birth almost killed her mother. A condition known as placenta praevia* caused her mum to haemorrhage and it was a miracle that mother and daughter survived.

Amanda's childhood was idyllic. She grew up in a beautiful seaside town called Moruya, a few hours' drive south of Sydney, with a population of around 3,000 people.

"I'm so lucky to have had such a lovely upbringing, where it was such a community. I would hug anybody in the street because I knew most of them, and it felt safe."

Opportunities for study and work were in short supply, and after finishing high school, Amanda left Moruya to study early childhood teaching in

Canberra. She graduated with her diploma after two years and found a job right away. It was quite a learning curve, especially as she had to fit into the centre's established methodology. She came in with fresh ideas and was judged to be emotional and weak. In contrast, Amanda saw her ability to build emotional connections with families as one of her strengths.

After work one day, a colleague was meeting up with her boyfriend and Amanda joined them for drinks. Call it luck, call it destiny, but her colleague's boyfriend was there with his brother, Jim who was visiting from Wollongong, a 2.5-hour drive away.

They exchanged numbers, and a couple of weeks later, Jim called Amanda and they started dating. Around eight months later, they decided that they wanted more than a long-distance relationship, so Amanda left her job and moved to Wollongong to be with Jim.

For seven years, they enjoyed a busy life, working and socialising with friends, hosting parties, going out and relishing time together as a young couple in their twenties. During those years, Amanda and her girlfriend Laura had often discussed participating in an overseas volunteer program.

One night over drinks, they decided to make their dream a reality. The two signed up and took off on a six-week trip to volunteer in an orphanage in Sri Lanka.

> **"It was incredible, a pivotal moment in my life. It was something I always wanted to do."**

Prior to leaving, Amanda's friends and colleagues expressed their concern over how she would cope.

> **"I was told I was so sad, so emotional. They said, 'You're not going to be able to survive. You'll be crying all the time. You're just not going to deal with this.' I just wanted to prove everybody wrong."**

Amanda not only coped, but she immersed herself in the culture. It opened her eyes and gave her a new perspective on the world.

> **"It was humbling to be around a culture that doesn't have much but gives a lot. Back here, we take so much for granted. We were on a long train ride, and there's this unspoken system where everybody sits down and takes a turn. They get up and someone else has a turn, and then they get up. Strangers will hold someone's baby for them because they've had enough. It's an absolutely incredible culture."**

At the orphanage, Amanda was initially dismayed by the lack of love and affection given to the children. She discovered that the staff held the belief that if they were given love, then they would want more love, so affection was discouraged. This philosophy was likely developed to avoid attachment as many of the workers were pregnant, unwed women who were there to give birth then leave their baby behind at the orphanage.

Amanda's training and 12 year of childcare experience had taught her that with love, children are more likely to explore and learn. She and Laura worked with the orphanage's toddlers aged from around two to four years and gave them the books and stickers they had brought over with them. The staff told them not to teach the children because they were too young to learn, but Amanda and Laura soon showed them that toddlers love to learn.

> **"By the time we left, we'd actually taught them lots of songs, and we taught the staff there as well. Those children needed me. I think we really did make a difference. Some of those children truly opened up while we were there."**

Amanda returned home, empowered by her incredible experience. She felt strong and capable, no longer the overemotional or sensitive person that others saw. The strangest thing was Jim's effusive declarations of love for her. He had missed her so much during those six weeks that he was motivated to arrange a welcome back party. Amanda's suspicions were aroused, and she had an inkling that something was up. Sure enough, at the party, in front of all their friends, Jim proposed.

The couple married the following year. Amanda was 29 and they settled into their new home. She decided that her 30th birthday would be her last hurrah before actively trying to start a family, and a couple of days after the party, Amanda discovered she was pregnant.

> **"It was so exciting to be pregnant. I had dreamt of that moment for ages because I'd always worked with children and thought about how nice it would be. I'd seen my sisters have babies and I'd helped with them, so I was fairly familiar with them."**

Amanda began journaling, documenting every step of her pregnancy. Together with Jim, they tracked the size of their baby and enjoyed all the special moments of planning and imagining what their child would be like. They decided not to find out the sex of the baby, but Amanda was convinced they were having a boy.

They prepared the nursery, choosing neutral greys and choosing unisex decorations. Amanda had some morning sickness but soon worked out that eating a dry cracker seemed to help. She had just started working at a new centre, and fortunately they were very supportive of her pregnancy. Her appetite escalated and she was eating everything, including the same meals that the children were eating!

Everything was progressing nicely. Jim and Amanda wanted to have a birth that was as natural as possible, so they prepared by attended a calm birth course. Amanda had massages and acupuncture. She did yoga and said her affirmations.

Amanda worked right up to 36 weeks, expecting to have four weeks to catch up with friends and prepare for the birth. She made it to her 38-week check which showed all was well. The baby's size was on track and she was told that bub was engaged. Amanda phoned her mum, a nurse by profession, and she got ready to make the drive up from Moruya.

The next day, Amanda had an exceptionally busy day planned. Her first appointment was with the acupuncturist, then she moved on to lunch with friends. That afternoon, Amanda noticed tightening pains in her tummy and felt a heaviness. The baby hadn't moved much all day, but she didn't stop to think about it at the time because she had to go straight out to a friend's birthday. By the time they got home it was around 9.30pm and even though Laura was staying over, she was too tired to chat and needed to lie down.

"I didn't feel the baby moving much. It wasn't concerning enough to go anywhere but I'd had these tightenings all day. I thought that maybe bub wasn't moving because they were in my birth canal. I just had this instinctive feeling that something was wrong, but I didn't want to be neurotic. I was a first-time mum and I didn't want to kick up a fuss because they said don't come in until the contractions start."

Jim asked if she wanted to go to hospital, but Amanda thought that she would go to bed and not worry because everything had been fine at her check-up the previous day.

"I woke up at one, and I just knew. I said to myself, 'There is nothing I can do right now. I'm just going to wake up in the morning and go in to the hospital.'"

As soon as she woke up, Amanda called the midwife who told her to come in immediately. Laura accompanied her to the birthing unit. The midwife searched and searched for a heartbeat with a doppler as Amanda held her breath. Then suddenly, they clicked onto a heartbeat. Her heart leapt but then sank as she realised it was her own.

The midwife told Amanda not to worry and that they would have a better look with an ultrasound. Deep down, she already knew. Her worst fears were confirmed with the scan.

> **"It was just an out-of-body experience at that point. I could hear this screaming, but I didn't know it was me that was screaming so much. It was just a really surreal experience from that point. Like slow motion. I felt really spaced out and I couldn't kind of concentrate on anything."**

Laura offered to call Jim. Amanda recalls instantly turning into a 'really calm machine' and called Jim herself. At this point, all she could think about was speaking as normally as possible to ensure Jim reached her safely. The minute he walked into the room and their eyes met, he knew and they both burst into tears.

The bereft couple left the hospital trying to process what had happened and to prepare for what was to come.

"We came home, and we just cried. We just sat in the nursery, which was all set up and ready to go and just cried for as long as it took."

They gathered up all the baby things from around their home and put everything into the nursery and closed the door. It was as if the weather reflected their emotional state—a storm had come over and the sky was all grey and gloomy. They decided to go for a walk down by the lake.

> **"At this point it was starting to rain, it was really cathartic. And again, this calmness came over me. I said, 'Well, I still get to have my baby, I just don't get to keep them. So, let's go and rock this.' And you know, I prepared for this moment, so there was no reason why I couldn't have it."**

The next day they went to stay at the hospital overnight before being induced in the morning. Amanda was in a single bed while Jim tried to sleep on a fold-out couch. It was awful. She was an emotional wreck, needing rest but unable to sleep.

> **"I just kept kind of howling like this crazy banshee. It actually felt like I was breaking in two. We got through the night, I don't**

know how, because we could hear babies in the corridor—it was awful."

Their midwife provided amazing care, preparing the couple for what was to come. She explained that the baby would have dark red lips and very fragile skin. She had also arranged for Heartfelt*, a volunteer organisation of professional photographers, to come in and take photos after the birth.

In the morning, the doctor inserted an IV* to induce labour. She discovered that the tightening pains she had experienced were actual contractions and she was already five centimetres dilated. Around six hours later, Eva Joyce arrived peacefully into the world.

"She was a girl! I was like, 'WHAT?!! It's a girl? I don't understand.' And I wasn't sure if I wanted to see her."

For Amanda, the birth was beautiful, peaceful and natural except for the induction. It was interesting when she later read back over her affirmation, that it didn't actually say anything about the baby breathing but had words about holding baby in her arms. That part came true.

The midwife wrapped Eva up and placed her in Amanda's arms. She was pretty and petite, so like Amanda as a baby. Fortunately, they had the use of a cuddle cot* that allowed time for family to meet her, and for the couple to spend lots of time cuddling and connecting with her. They read to Eva, just as they had when she was inside Amanda's tummy.

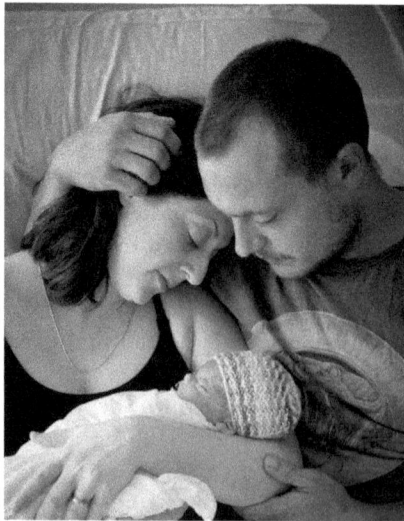

Amanda and Jim with Eva

Not knowing whether their baby was going to be a boy or a girl, the couple had only packed plain white clothing. Amanda smiled as she remembered dressing Eva and looking down at her, thinking that her gorgeous girl looked like she was about to do judo—she looked ridiculous! A pretty beanie from the staff soon fixed that.

"Seeing her was surreal. I've never seen Jim cry like that. He was so upset. It just gutted us because we had come to this point, you know, it's nine months of preparing for something."

It was also difficult for Amanda's father, seeing his youngest daughter having to deal with the loss. Her mum, as a nurse and through her own experiences as a mother, was better equipped to handle the situation and provided much appreciated support.

Amanda received excellent care, except for a comment made by one of the registrars following the birth. He said, "Oh, this is so rare. You know, the odds of this happening are so small."

"We felt super alienated by that. It wasn't until later that we discovered that it happens every day."

Around lunchtime the following day, the couple felt that it was the right time to leave. They cherished the 24 hours they spent with Eva and wanted to leave at a top point—if it had been any more it would have been too hard to bear.

"I don't know how we survived, honestly. The days after that were actually horrific. I don't think I've cried that much in my life and I don't think I've hurt so much in my life and my heart cavity hurt. It was like this constant heaviness sitting on my chest. I didn't sleep very well. We ate like crap and both took sleeping tablets to try and get some sleep. Every time we turned the TV on, there'd be a baby and I thought, 'Is this some kind of sick joke?' So, we sat there, sort of just being with each other, just hugging."

These awful days were brightened by friends popping in to visit and celebrate their wedding anniversary. It helped to pull them out of a terrible place where they questioned everything. Amanda could not help thinking, 'Why me? Why us? What did I do wrong?' Jim felt it was some sort of penance. But friends helped them connect back with life. At some points, Amanda felt that she would never smile or laugh again, but one of their friends, known for his sense of humour, dropped in and had them laughing at his jokes. It gave them hope that they could survive their loss.

The shared trauma bonded Jim and Amanda as a couple. It made them stronger together, even though they dealt with their grief differently. Amanda is the kind of woman who wears her heart on her sleeve, and when her friends asked if she was okay, she would tell them exactly how she felt. Since then, her friends have told her that it was awesome that she was able to express her true feelings because it made them feel more connected to her in the moment. It allowed them to be there for her.

Amanda recalls Eva's funeral as an incredible day. That morning, she was again struck by overwhelming calm, making a memory book of Eva. She managed to get through her whole speech without crying, and it was only when Jim carried the coffin that she broke down. They recorded it all on video, but she has not watched it, and is unsure if she ever will.

Amanda is a fixer, so a few weeks later, she knew she had to change something. She read books, researched online, and realised that this type of loss is part of life and that people get through it. Amanda started chatting to people on forums and then discovered a local support group.

> **"It was so powerful to know these people. They're strangers, but I felt more connected to them than I had to anyone for a long time. We shared the same heartache and it's indescribable. When you don't have to describe it to anyone, you just relax, and you get to just be."**

At their six-week check, the couple received Eva's autopsy results. It revealed that her small placenta and the early contractions were the likely causes of her passing. The condition is called placenta chronic villitis* and in Amanda's case, it spread like wildfire causing her placenta to die.

The worst thing for Amanda was that the doctor could not tell her if the condition was hereditary or if it would happen again. She was really scared and searched for information on the internet. That made it worse. She started to think that she would never have children again.

> **"I even said to Jim, 'I don't mind if you want to leave me because I can't give you babies.' He said, 'Don't be stupid. Your next pregnancy will be different.' He is a good man, he's an incredible man."**

Once Jim went back to work, Amanda felt unhappy about the changes that pregnancy had made to her body. She had excess weight and skin and even though she had taken a tablet to stop breast milk production, she still had milk. It felt unfair, having all these physical symptoms and no baby.

She decided to become the healthiest person she could be, eating well and running every day. Amanda developed a daily ritual to keep herself on track. She would get up in the morning, eat a healthy breakfast, light a candle for Eva and go on her run down by the lakeside where Eva was buried. It gave her a routine and a great way to start off the day.

Other activities that helped Amanda heal included regular counselling sessions to assist her mental health and also taking Franchesca Cox's course on the facets of grief. Amanda believes that her willingness to articulate her feelings brought them out into the open so that she could better analyse what lay under the surface of her emotions.

After a few months, Amanda felt ready to return to work part-time. Thankfully, her workplace offered her an office role rather than her previous position on the floor as a teacher. It was perfect—the new position upskilled her into a trainer and assessor.

Amanda moved forward, one day at a time. Then, after about three months postpartum, she found out she was pregnant.

> **"The pregnancy was anxiety-filled of course. I was still stuck in this grief as well. I didn't really connect very much with the baby. I was still stuck in my light the candle, go out, go for a walk, go to work. Things got busy, and I hadn't had a chance to connect until the baby started moving. Then I realised, this is real. Every scan, I'm hyperventilating. I'm thinking, I can't do this. What if this baby dies too? I would be holding on to every movement and I'd be really tight in my chest."**

It took some strong words from her midwife to help her to get her mind out of the past and into the present. She said that Amanda was a wonderful mum for Eva, but that she needed to wake up and be present for the baby inside her. Her words hit the mark and shook Amanda hard. She thought, "Okay I've got this. I'm going to do this." Amanda reminded herself that this was a different pregnancy and developed her mindfulness practice, focussing on being present in the moment.

Amanda felt that she needed to change anything that was in Eva's pregnancy. She didn't do acupuncture or massage therapy. She ate different foods. But at night, when everything was still, anxiety would hit, and she would poke her belly until the baby moved.

As her due date approached, Amanda didn't want to reach the 38 weeks because that's when she lost Eva. She insisted that the baby be delivered at

37.5 weeks even though there were no signs of labour. To make this happen, her doctor inserted a Foley bulb* to open her cervix. The other issue that had to be solved was that the baby was not engaged and still in a high position.

> **"Don't mess with me, I'm a lioness. I said, 'This baby's coming out.' Someone was pushing on me while I broke my water. That was the most painful thing I've ever had in my life. When it came time for crowning, the baby would come out and go back in. Out and in for about an hour. It was excruciating. Then they finally pulled her out and it was pretty intense. She wasn't ready, not anywhere near ready."**

Lilian arrived gurgling until they cleared her airways. Everything stopped. Amanda was freaked out until she heard her baby cry.

> **"And then I was like, what do I do with it now? I have no idea. This is so weird. And I was sobbing, absolutely sobbing."**

Amanda had developed gestational diabetes during her pregnancy. She was just on the cusp and her doctor suggested later that this might have been the cause of Lilian's poor blood sugar levels, resulting in the newborn being whisked away to for special care.

> **"It was really scary. That was probably the scariest thing, not being able to have her, keep her, and I was really anxious."**

The new parents were taken to see their baby, and they were wanted to stay with their newborn daughter. For some reason the NICU staff would not allow them to stay, sending Jim home and Amanda back to the maternity ward. Amanda remembers it as an awful, lonely night.

Due to her blood sugar readings, Amanda was taken up to special care every two hours to feed Lilian. The newborn was woken for feeds then woken again for injections and Amanda feels that these constant interruptions contributed to Lilian developing unsettled sleep patterns. The nurses were also topping her up with formula and this was incredibly traumatic for Amanda, watching her baby vomit it up.

The formula was given to provide extra milk so they did not have to increase Lilian's dose of sugar syrup, but it was a waste of time because she would bring it back up. Amanda asked them to stop, but they just kept on feeding her with formula, saying something else was wrong with her.

> **"A registrar came up to me and asked, 'What did your last baby die of?' I said, 'Nothing. What is wrong has nothing to do with that.' And she said, 'I'm going to have to ultrasound or x-ray her belly because we think something's wrong.' At that point, I lost it. The paediatrician finally came and touched her belly, saying, 'Nothing's wrong. Just stop giving her formula.'"**

Amanda pumped like a 'jersey cow' to show them that she could provide enough milk for her baby. Then they diagnosed Lilian with jaundice and she was placed under special lights for two days. By this time, Amanda was so sick of not being in the same room with her baby that she threatened to discharge both of them, so they found her a private room.

Because of the jaundice, the staff wanted to start supplementing with formula again.

> **"I said, 'No, you're not.' I was bawling. I had two pumps going and my midwife came down and said, 'Listen to her.' I was honestly over it. It was really traumatic to me. I was going crazy and just wanted to go home."**

A week later, the family finally went home together. A couple of weeks before Lilian's birth, they had opened the nursery. They looked at the walls and realised they had decorated it with rainbows. That was kind of freaky, as the room was going to be for their rainbow baby.

The first three months of parenthood were tough for Jim and Amanda. Lilian had silent reflux* and her sleep times were all over the place.

> **"I'd be rocking her on the chair at one o'clock in the morning going, 'What have I done? I've wanted this baby for two years and now I don't know if I can do this.' I talked to my psychologist and she said, 'Normal mothers feel like that, but you've got this whole other ballgame of grief going on.' I said, 'Yeah, I just felt like I deserved an easy child after I've gone through all this stuff.'"**

It is two years on now, and Lilian is a busy and articulate toddler. This year, Jim and Amanda felt that the time was right to add to their family. A pregnancy in February 2019 ended in miscarriage at six weeks, and another in June was lost at eight weeks. These two losses made Amanda seek answers.

> **"It just didn't make sense to me. One, I can deal with, but two? Really? Is that what we're doing now? Am I going to be one of**

those women that has to be learning through every gestational loss? Maybe I'm supposed to have one of every type so I can help all these women in the world."

Life may not be fair, but Amanda's experiences have equipped her to help many. She has successfully fundraised to purchase a cuddle cot for Bowral Hospital. She is also an active member of the Illawarra Baby and Child Loss Community and the co-organiser of their annual 'Remember Me' Bridge Walk for Babies. Amanda does it for Eva, for her daughter's legacy, and it brings her immense joy.

At the time of writing, Amanda is 20 weeks pregnant. She is stronger, wiser and a little more serene. She feels that the world keeps wanting to teach her the lesson that control is an illusion. And even though those dark thoughts still creep in, she is happy in her skin this pregnancy, and hopeful for the future.

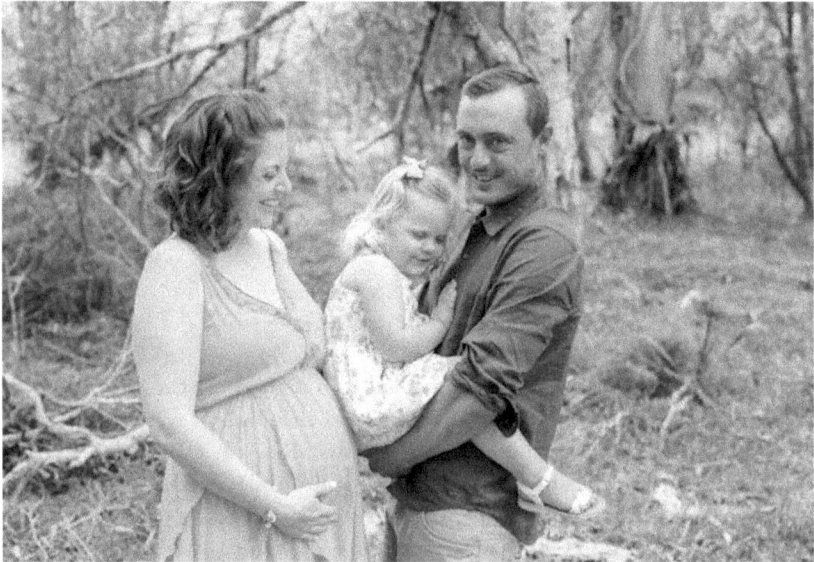

Amanda, Lillian and Jim

"I still have like days where I am on a roller-coaster of emotions, when I feel things getting stressful or upsetting. I'm human. But later, I can kind of reflect back on things and go, okay, well what do I need to do from here to get myself centred again? So, I'd journal my feelings, write letters to Eva and my future self. I do all of these things."

8

KAZ

- Professional Midwife
- Facet Joint* injury
- Bicornuate Uterus*
- Tarl, aged 20
- Toran, aged 15

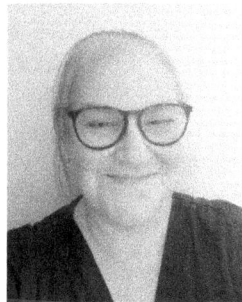

Kaz has been a dear friend for close to 25 years. She has a natural consideration for the well-being of others, so it is no wonder that she chose nursing, and specifically midwifery, as a profession. It is an arena where her traits of empathy and kindness are highly valued by the women she cares for.

When Kaz started her nursing diploma after high school, she embarked on a course that was split equally between university learning and practical hospital experience in the Royal North Shore Hospital, Sydney.

> **"It was designed to give you a smorgasbord of experiences. As soon as I saw my first birth, I felt that I had to be part of that. It was definitely the area I wanted to work in. So the very next year, after I finished my nursing degree, I started midwifery."**

Now, with more than 30 years of experience as a professional midwife, Kaz reflected on the comparative simplicity of the process of getting the same qualification today.

"It took six years for me to become a midwife. Now you can do it by direct entry. You don't even have to be a nurse."

Her midwifery training was held at the Royal Women's Hospital, Sydney, established in 1820 and still regarded as one of Australia's foremost specialist hospitals for women and babies. It was a brilliant place to learn from the country's best doctors and midwives operating in both a traditional labour ward and a birth centre in a separate cottage.

After achieving her qualification, Kaz continued to work there for 10 years. I asked her to share her most memorable experiences.

"Probably one of the best was when friends of mine who had been trying to have a baby for years, and years and years finally got pregnant. And I was actually on duty the day they came in to have the baby. I got to deliver the baby and just be with them. That was very satisfying and magical and amazing and tear-jerking. Pretty much, any birth that's not dramatic is amazing. The dramatic ones, it's just stressful. But most births, women could do it without any help really. They just need a bit of mental and emotional support."

Through her work, Kaz met several home birth midwives who were accredited to the hospital. She noticed that they had a good relationship with the doctors and the hospital, confident that if anything went wrong, they could bring their women in for assistance.

As a self-confessed hippie and an advocate for natural therapies, the concept of home birth was very appealing. While working full-time, Kaz added to her skillset by doing a home birth apprenticeship so that she could assist women who made that choice.

When she was in her early thirties, Kaz met her husband Dave. He was eight years older than her and already had a stepdaughter from his first marriage, but no children of his own.

"When Dave and I got together, he never thought he'd have more children, but it was his absolute dream. I was 33 and said, 'Okay, let's give it a go.' And the second month off the pill I got pregnant."

At around seven weeks gestation, just a week after she discovered she was pregnant, Kaz suffered a serious work injury.

"I was helping a woman to give birth and her foot was on my pelvis. That's how we used to do it. One foot came onto my hip and the other foot was on the doctor's hip. As the baby came out, the woman pulled her leg back and kicked me in the pelvis and I collapsed."

She felt like the kick had broken something in her back and she was unable to get up. Due to her pregnancy, they were not able to do an x-ray, so Kaz was sent to a neurologist. His best diagnosis was that she probably had a damaged facet joint in her spine. This evaluation was subsequently verified as a permanent injury.

Placed on workers' compensation by her employer, Kaz was given leave to heal from her injury. Around the same time, she also decided to hire an independent midwife to look after her throughout her pregnancy.

"I wanted someone who was just there for me, no matter what. I wanted a home birth because I was petrified of the hospital."

Knowing that Kaz had spent most of her working life in hospitals, I asked her for clarification. She explained that she'd seen things that she didn't agree with such as cases when medical staff insisted a woman should have a caesarean, or decisions to induce if a woman didn't go into labour by a certain time. Kaz wanted her birth to be without interference and with the control that a home birth offered.

"If you have a midwife who knows what they are doing, they're never going to put you in a situation of harm because their number one priority is your safety."

The couple hired Marie, a rural midwife who had worked as the head of a hospital maternity unit before she became a home birth midwife. If something did go wrong, Kaz had confidence in Marie's judgement and the assurance that the hospital was only five minutes away.

Kaz's pregnancy continued without incident apart from a small bleed at around 14 weeks that resolved itself. During the final weeks of gestation, Kaz walked along the beach every day and wrote in a journal that she had started on the day she discovered she was pregnant. The baby's due date passed and a week later, her waters broke.

"They broke at five o'clock in the morning and there was a slight tinge of yellowy green. I thought it could be meconium*."

Kaz did not panic, she had seen similar in other women before and as her labour began she contacted Marie who happened to be delivering another baby some distance away. Dave filled up the birthing pool and Kaz went into the pool.

Labour stopped, and she got out of the pool. Kaz's mother and sister came over to help and Marie also arrived later that day, her checks confirming that the baby was in the breech position. Kaz's on and off labour ended up continuing for two days.

> **"We had a monitor on the baby's heart rate, we were checking my temperature and doing everything right. I didn't want to go to the hospital, but Marie said, 'Kaz, it's not about you anymore. It's really safety first. Sometimes babies come out this way, you know that.' I was so devastated."**

On reflection, Kaz realised that she had a specific vision of how she wanted her baby to be born.

> **"It was all ego driven. I thought, 'I'm going to show everyone how great home birth is. I can do it.' But parenting and birth, it's all such a teaching lesson, isn't it? It was telling me to surrender and let go."**

They went into hospital and had an ultrasound. The sonographer told them that the baby was 4.5kg, a huge size despite her being overdue. Kaz highly doubted that was true. What the scan did reveal was that she had a bicornuate uterus and this was probably the reason the baby was in the breech position. It meant that she would have to have a caesarean section.

After two hours of monitoring, Kaz was told that she needed to have a caesarean by general anaesthetic.

> **"They said, 'You've waited long enough. We're not doing an epidural now.' That was their exact words."**

Kaz was prepared for surgery and all she remembers is someone pushing her midwife out of the way as they shoved a mask on her face and wheeled her into theatre. When she woke in the recovery ward, she was alone without her baby. Confused and distressed, she questioned the nurse.

> **"I asked, 'Where's my baby?' I had said to Dave, 'Don't leave the baby. Don't let anyone do anything. Don't let them give any needles, don't let them do anything without my permission.' He was the guardian of our baby."**

Dave followed their newborn son, Tarl to the NICU. He weighed a healthy 3.8kg but was still given oxygen and a drip. Kaz desperately wanted to see her baby but was taken to the ward and told that they were really busy and didn't have any wheelchairs.

"Normally you would take a mother on her bed to see her baby. But there was none of that. I pressed the buzzer and kept buzzing, buzzing and buzzing. I was beside myself. Honestly, all I could think about was seeing him. It was an overwhelming need to see him, so I just got up and walked."

Tarl was in a humidicrib on oxygen to assist his breathing, but otherwise, he was fine. Kaz took him out of his hospital gown, dressed him in a cute little tie-dyed jumpsuit and added a couple of healing crystals to his crib.

Within 24 hours, Tarl was out of the humidicrib, breastfeeding well and Kaz discharged them both from hospital.

In comparison, Kaz's second pregnancy was planned and scheduled. It was five years later and during that time she had developed a persistent cough that she is still battling some 15 years later.

"I was worried about the cough, so I had three scans during the pregnancy. At the 20-week scan, the ultrasonographer gasped, and I said, 'What's wrong?' What a stupid thing for her to do. Just don't do that to a woman. She said, 'I've never seen a baby do this. It's doing the splits. There's one leg up around the head and the other leg is straight down.'"

The baby was also in a breech position. At 36 weeks, Kaz went to have acupuncture to turn the baby around. It worked, but soon after, the baby returned to the breech position. They tried three times with the same result.

With the knowledge gained from her previous delivery, Kaz knew that with her bicornuate uterus and the baby's breech position, it meant that she was more likely to need a caesarean. In preparation, she booked a private obstetrician and anaesthetist for an elective caesarean.

It was as if this baby decided to mirror the initial stages of Tarl's birth. Kaz's waters broke at the exact same time—5am, one week after the baby's due date. But this time it contained thick black meconium and she knew they needed to get to the hospital immediately.

"It was so much better. I had my epidural, but I was petrified. The epidural was the scariest thing in my whole life. Just the

thought of the needle going into my back...I don't even like watching them."

The epidural was a success and for Kaz, her second delivery was much calmer. She was so happy to be awake to experience her baby's birth.

"It was a lovely elective caesarean. The only thing that happened that was weird was that an intern fainted. He was holding the clamps as part of the operation and as he fainted, I could feel everything sort of pull and I'm like, 'Let go of the clamp!'"

Toran was born and placed straight onto Kaz's chest. Despite the meconium, he did not have any respiratory issues. Now 15 years of age, he is fulfilling the potential he signalled when he was doing the splits at 20 weeks in utero—Toran is a hip-hop dancer competing and winning dance competitions!

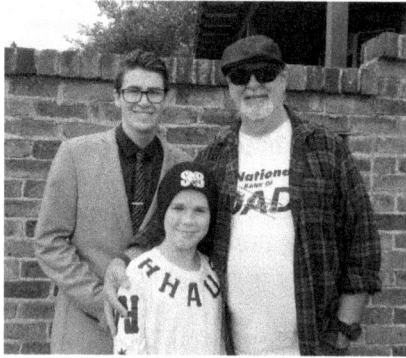

Dave with sons Tarl and Toran

While raising her boys, Kaz decided to take a break from hospital midwifery to start her own business from home. She is thriving in her success as she continues to grow it further. Kaz has expanded her expertise to teaching birthing classes privately and is now also conducting group classes for hospitals.

From her many years of helping women through pregnancy and birth, I asked Kaz for tips to help couples prepare for their birthing experience.

"Labour is going to be hard work. If you're her partner, then you have to be her coach. If you don't think you can do that, let her know so she can get someone who can. Because she needs

eye contact. She needs to be told she can do it. You need to be able to watch her when she's not breathing and she's holding tight, just to remind her to drop her shoulders and breathe in and out, so her energy is flowing.

In my classes, I say to have a code word. If you don't say the code word, even if you look like you're in a lot of pain, no one in your support team will offer you pain relief because it's undermining your personal power. If you do say the code word, then you'll get pain relief, no questions asked, not, 'Are you sure you need it?' Code word means drop everything, get pain relief. And no code word means, support her and tell her she'd doing a fantastic job."

For women who have experienced miscarriage loss, the joy of pregnancy can be overwhelmed by fear and anxiety. Though Kaz has not experienced this herself, she lived through the fear felt by her sister whose pregnancy was almost two weeks overdue.

"She was petrified. I wanted to write her some affirmations to remind her that her body was strong and could birth her baby. That everything was going to be alright. When I gave them to her, it really helped her. The point of them was to get rid of fear, be at peace, to have some joy and be in the moment."

Kaz realised that these affirmations could help many women. Together with her friend and artist Gabbi, she created a beautiful book of affirmations called "Sweet Surrender" for women either trying to get pregnant or who are already pregnant. The book is available from her www.sweetsurrender.com.au website where you can also access her personal and online birthing classes.

"It's a sacred space. Bringing a new life into the world is a pure, magical miracle. You are privileged to be there, to be part of helping it happen and empowering the woman to push through and transcend her own fears.

And then at the end, this tiny little new bit of him, and new bit of her come out. And if it's a same sex couple, it's the same magical feeling. We are all the same, love for our new child is so special. And they don't even look if it's a boy or a girl. It's just this being, this new human being that they're part of. And it's just amazing."

9

KRYSTIN

- Endometriosis*
- One Miscarriage
- Rainbow baby Mia, aged seven, Reflux
- Four Miscarriages
- Rainbow baby Willow, aged two

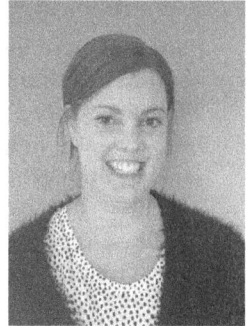

McDonald's Restaurants may be known for their fast food, but for Krystin and Matt, they hold a more significant meaning—working in the same restaurant brought them together. Krystin was just 17 years old and had known Matt's twin sister at school, but it wasn't until they started serving fries and Big Macs that the romance sparked!

Their mutual desire to travel led to holidays in their dream destinations including Europe, Thailand, Fiji and Queensland. Matt was studying at the time, and it was convenient for the couple to base themselves at Krystin's parents' place. As retirees, her parents were frequently away on adventures in their caravan so having their home occupied worked out well for everyone.

Life was going well until Krystin began experiencing abnormal pain before and during her periods. She was 24 years old, and the frequency of the pain just didn't seem right so Krystin decided to see her GP.

"He kind of made out that I was not experiencing anything, that everybody gets period pain. I was quite put off, I felt like

he wasn't taking me seriously. I thought, 'I'm not attention seeking, I need to have this checked.'"

The doctor reluctantly arranged a laparoscopy* to investigate and when Krystin returned to learn her results, the doctor apologised for doubting her. He said it was obvious why she was in pain. Krystin's bowel was stuck to her uterus and her ovaries were stuck to each other. She was diagnosed with Stage 3 Endometriosis and booked in for surgery to remove the displaced endometrial tissue.

Following her successful operation, Krystin's doctor asked if she had thought about having children. With her condition, he warned that she may have difficulty conceiving later in life. He suggested that now was the best time to conceive easily, while her reproductive organs were clear of tissue.

The doctor's advice caused the couple to try for a baby earlier than they had anticipated. From what they had been told, they expected to fall pregnant fairly quickly. One month passed, two, three and Krystin started to wonder why she wasn't pregnant.

"You don't really notice until you are in the situation of trying to have a baby. You're seeing people pregnant all the time. You're seeing babies all the time. It really heightens your awareness of pregnancy and babies. It was a struggle because I just thought it would be easy and it wasn't. We were so young, so it was hard, it became a chore to try."

It did put a little stress on their relationship, mostly due to their differences in personality. Krystin is the type of person who is impatient to get things done. She is grateful that Matt is easy going and that "nothing really phases fazes him."

Having been together for almost eight years at this stage, they knew each other really well and were able to understand that it was the situation that was creating the tension.

Around 11 months after they started trying, the young couple was thrilled to discover that they were pregnant! This happy event happened just before Krystin was scheduled to go with a friend for a psychic reading. She estimates she was about six weeks pregnant and expectantly anticipated hearing something about her pregnancy, but the psychic did not mention it. On the way home, her friend was excited to share that the psychic had told her she was pregnant.

"I said, 'Oh, are you?' and my friend said 'Yes, I am.' I said, 'I am too, but she didn't say anything to me.' We worked out that our due dates were two days apart, so I was freaking out."

Krystin tried to put it all in perspective, after all, psychics aren't always right. The two pregnant friends were the first in their group to fall pregnant, so they were excited to be sharing the experience with each other and their partners.

Later that week, Krystin's joy was disrupted by bleeding. Her mum accompanied her to the imaging centre for an ultrasound and Krystin recalls how upset the experience made her feel.

"He was a male sonographer and really insensitive actually. It was an internal examination and while that was still happening, he said, 'This baby's not alive. You're gonna lose this baby.' It was a horrible situation, the way it happened, the way he said it."

And that was the end of the appointment. The sonographer failed to check with the radiographer for an expert second opinion, he just sent them on their way.

Krystin tried to remain calm, telling herself it was going to be fine. They went straight to their doctor who agreed that it was early. He asked her to do a blood test and to go back for another ultrasound in a week's time.

"That week was just hell. I went to work, and I just couldn't do anything. I couldn't concentrate, I just felt sick. My doctor was saying that the test might be wrong. He was giving me hope, false hope."

Krystin held onto that hope, convincing herself that the doctor was right and that everything would be fine. Matt accompanied her to the next ultrasound where Krystin requested a female sonographer. After her last experience, she definitely did not want to be scanned by a male.

Looking back, Krystin realises how naïve she was at the time. The sonographer's silence made her think that everything was okay. The couple waited all day for the images and then took them directly to the doctor. He examined the scans and informed them that their baby had no heartbeat and had shrunk in size. That was their first miscarriage.

"I was sent to my obstetrician and had a D & C within the week. It was a really crap couple of weeks from finding out my

baby was dead, then hopeful, and then wondering if I was going to lose it naturally before surgery."

Krystin was gutted. She never considered it a possibility that this could happen to her. Why did it happen? What did she do wrong? These were the questions that plagued her. Up to that point in her life, this was the most traumatic event Krystin had ever experienced and she was angry, sad and devastated.

One of the most difficult things for Krystin to cope with during this time was the pregnancy announcements of friends and siblings. When she read a Facebook post announcing that their nephew would be a big brother, Krystin cried uncontrollably. Friends would text to say they were pregnant, and she would dissolve in a flood of tears. Seeing her friend having a healthy pregnancy and growing bigger each week was especially hard— Krystin could not help but think that that should have been her experience. These happy events acted as triggers, reminding Krystin of her loss.

"They would try and ring me and I didn't want to speak to them. I was happy for them, but I was jealous, I was angry that it wasn't me, I was sad for myself. I remember getting up in the middle of the night and crying in the bathroom, thinking, 'Why is she having a baby? She's already got a baby and now she's having another one...' I would just cry and cry and cry. I just couldn't stop myself crying. I've never been so low than at those times."

Throughout her emotional turmoil, Matt was an unwavering support. If he was apart from Krystin when they received a pregnancy announcement from a friend, Matt would ring her immediately and ask, "Are you OK?" Krystin's mum was also a tower of strength, holding her and just being there when she needed the hugs.

Krystin had a D & C, and due to the length of time it took for her to conceive the first time, the doctor prescribed Clomid*, an ovulatory stimulating drug used to help women who have problems with ovulation.

A few weeks later, Krystin's pop passed away, adding to her sense of loss. So, the couple decided to take a complete break before trying to conceive again. They left for a week of total relaxation in Fiji.

The need for a dramatic life change would serve as a way for Krystin to put a 'full-stop' on her current experience so that she could move forward. The complete break served its purpose and Krystin felt emotionally ready to try again.

The Clomid worked wonders and Krystin was ecstatic to find out she was pregnant in the first month!

"I was so excited but full of anxiety that it would happen again."

They went to the seven-week scan with great trepidation. It was an immense relief to see the baby measuring perfectly with a beautiful heartbeat. The pregnancy continued progressing normally and at 39 weeks, Krystin's obstetrician said that with women who had experienced fertility issues, it was best not to go past their due date. He also mentioned he was going away for the weekend, so Krystin is unsure if the decision to deliver was motivated by medical or personal reasons! Either way, she was happy to be induced. After a nine-hour labour, an epidural and the help of a vacuum extractor, Mia Louise was brought into the world.

"My mum was a great support during labour. I asked her to come in, but she said this was just for me and Matt. She waited there all day, and my dad came later after a funeral he had to attend. There was no one else in the delivery room suite so when they heard a baby cry, they were so excited!"

Krystin was especially grateful for the support of her mum during the first few weeks home with Mia. Breastfeeding proved to be a big challenge so Krystin expressed milk until Mia was six weeks old. By that time, she made the difficult decision to put Mia on the bottle as her milk supply could not keep up with her baby's demands.

Mia developed reflux, and this meant that she was difficult to settle and would cry day and night. It was a massive physical and emotional challenge for the new parents.

"I did struggle a bit with her. I don't think I got postnatal depression, but I did have my ups and downs. Looking back, it was probably that I was a new mum, I didn't know what I was doing. No one would give me any medication to help her with the reflux until she was nine months old. So, for nine months, she screamed, she didn't sleep, it was a tough time. We hardly slept."

It was so bad that the exhausted parents sought help from their GP, only to be told that Mia was behaving like any normal baby. This conclusion was probably due to the fact that their baby was angelically sleeping for the duration of the doctor's visit. Krystin asked for a referral to a specialist paediatrician, explaining that Mia was sleeping now because she had not slept all night. The GP said that there was no need and they were sent home, frustrated by their inability get the help they so desperately needed. Krystin was also disappointed with the support from the baby health clinic.

"I think they are quite intimidating. When they come into the home for the first visit, they are all very judgemental, focusing on domestic violence and looking for something to be wrong. I understand that's important, but I thought, 'Where's the support for me?' I found them very unapproachable."

It was a blessing that Krystin's parents could to assist with caring for Mia. When she was around the age of one, the couple decided to sell their home to purchase a house and land package. While waiting for their new home to be built, the young family moved in with Krystin's parents.

This move allowed Krystin to go back to work, three days a week. The financial saving was beneficial, but it was difficult to adjust to being back in the family home with a daughter of their own. They did, however, manage to make it work.

Motherhood turned out to be different to what Krystin had envisaged.

"I'd always thought I would be this really great mother. I loved babies, always wanted babies and couldn't wait to be a mum. Then when it happened, I thought, 'I'm just not cut out for this. It's just not me.'"

Those first two years of Mia's life were really challenging, but by the time she was two, Mia began sleeping a little better. There is the myth that women are biologically programmed to forget the pain of childbirth and the first few weeks of parenting a newborn. This thinking is not scientifically proven, but there is much anecdotal evidence of this occurring. Perhaps it is not so much that the pain is forgotten, but that happiness and reward colours our memories.

This was the case with Krystin. Mia was such a cute child, a real character, that she let go of all those early dramas with Mia and within a few weeks Krystin was pregnant.

"When I found out, I was really happy. I didn't even think of miscarriage. I thought, 'Great! There must have been something wrong with the first baby, that happens.'"

At the first scan, the couple were told that their baby measured a week behind, just a few millimetres. This was explained away with wrong conception dates and Krystin felt that it was a logical explanation because her periods were so erratic. They saw a heartbeat, the same as with Mia, so they thought that everything would work out.

The weekend before the 12-week scan, Krystin and Matt were meant to attend a friend's birthday. On the Saturday morning Krystin started bleeding and automatically thought the worst. Her parents researched online and told her not to worry, perhaps it was a breakthrough bleed.

They did not want to take any chances and decided to go directly to hospital. Krystin has A negative blood type and she knew that any bleed meant that she had to have an Anti-D immunoglobulin injection. This medication prevents her body from forming antibodies, protecting her future pregnancies.

Krystin was given the injection and put on a drip. The nurse took her in for an ultrasound, and the scan revealed that the baby did not have a heartbeat. From what they could see, the baby had died a couple of weeks after the last ultrasound.

It was diagnosed as a missed miscarriage, where the baby dies but the body does not expel the tissue.

> **"I was devastated. That was harder than the first time because I'd seen a heartbeat and thought everything was okay, and then it wasn't. So, we were thinking, 'How did that happen?' It was different to my last experience."**

The experience was different, but it bought back all the emotions Krystin had experienced after her first miscarriage.

> **"I was crying for days. I just couldn't comprehend it. This was much harder. With the first one, I could understand that it happens, but now I know I can carry a baby."**

Krystin went into hospital a few days later for her scheduled D & C. Coincidentally, the timing couldn't have been worse—she was admitted at the same time as a friend was giving birth.

As with her previous experience, Krystin closed off that chapter of her life with another big change. This time, the family of three moved into their beautiful new home. For the next few months, they kept busy with decorating and landscaping while they healed from their loss.

Around four months later, Krystin felt ready to try again. The Clomid worked its magic and she fell pregnant during the second month. The combination of joy and anxiety began again. Krystin chose a different imagining centre that only used women for pregnancy ultrasounds and attended her seven-week scan.

The baby measured a week behind and this pregnancy mirrored her previous miscarriage—at 12 weeks they found that the baby had stopped growing at nine weeks. Krystin was plunged into absolute devastation.

> **"My feelings definitely got worse every pregnancy because it went from being normal to have one or two miscarriages to now being on my third. I would google percentages and this miscarriage put me in a small two percent group of women who experience what I did. I was grasping for anything and it did my head in. I was a mess. I just needed something to hold onto, because there was nothing else. I kept thinking there was something wrong with me."**

Even though Krystin was booked in for a D & C the next day, that night she had constant contractions and bleeding. She rang the doctors and was told to "just let it happen, only go to hospital if you really have to." Krystin did not miscarry naturally, she still had to go through with the procedure the next day.

To help her recovery from her latest loss, this time Krystin decided to bring a puppy into their lives. Rosie is a replacement for her lost babies, and she is now a much-loved member of the family.

Krystin's third miscarriage did not deter her from trying again. She was totally focussed on her wish to have another child in the family and the couple tried to conceive again a few months later. Again, she fell pregnant quickly. At her seven-week ultrasound, the sonographer said, "You're due on Christmas Day, what a shame!" Krystin was taken aback as she was happy to take any day at that point! The sonographer began moving the wand, and then suddenly stopped. Krystin knew that look, she had seen it before—the sonographer told her that the baby had no heartbeat.

Again, Krystin had her D & C and escaped to her happy place—watching reality tv on the lounge. It had become her coping mechanism, disappearing into someone else's tv life so that she could stop thinking about herself for a while.

Once she recovered, she decided to take matters into her own hands. Thinking that she needed to be fitter and healthier to carry her babies to term, Krystin embarked a new lifestyle of exercise, healthy eating, meditation and acupuncture.

When she thinks about that period of her life, Krystin acknowledges that a key factor in her ability to recover after each miscarriage was the support of her family and close friends. Matt was always understanding, her parents accompanied her to appointments when Matt could not, and they were always there to babysit Mia.

Something that stands out for Krystin is the way that her best friend, aunties and cousin showed their support. They were not intrusive or overbearing, nor did they disappear and ignore her. They struck just the right balance by dropping in with little gifts like flowers, chocolates and brownies. They would ask her out to dinner or coffee, just as an excuse to get Krystin out of the house. Their thoughtfulness helped to get her mind off her grief. They would call and text regularly, just enough to let her know that they were there and that they cared.

This support and her own determination to continue fuelled Krystin's desire to try again. She went back onto the Clomid and unexpectedly, did not fall pregnant straight away.

"I was worried, thinking that I'm a bit older, I am damaged and have scar tissue."

Krystin did eventually fall pregnant, finding out around her 30th birthday celebrations. She was in that awkward position of not drinking, and not wanting to explain why. Everything appeared normal at the first scan, but by the 12-week scan, her doctor found that there was no heartbeat.

"It was emotion, on emotion, on emotion. It was really starting to bring me down. My personality was changing. I was becoming bitter. I would lash out at my husband because I was feeling so sad and angry. Friends were having their second and third babies and I was jealous, I didn't want to be around them. I'm normally such a social person, I love people, I love socialising and I didn't want to."

I asked Krystin how she got out of that dark place. She said it was her Dad that made all the difference. He is experienced with grief and Post-Traumatic Stress Disorder (PTSD), and he was able help her see things differently. He pointed out that Krystin and Matt were putting their lives on hold in this desperation to have another child. He gave her some much-needed perspective, saying that he noticed that they weren't really enjoying Mia. He helped Krystin to see that Mia was getting older and if she didn't change things, she would miss out on this important time with her because she was so focussed on having another baby. This really struck a chord with Krystin, and it pulled her out of her grief.

"Dad reminded me to be grateful for what I had. He made me realise that I have to enjoy Mia because life's too short. I've had her, and it's not her fault that I'm losing these babies. She's missing out on having her mum."

This helped Krystin to bring balance back into her life. She cherished the summer break with Mia and her parents down on the South Coast.

They made the decision to try again, but with a new plan. Her miscarried baby was tested, and Krystin and Matt were tested too. Everything was normal. So, their obstetrician referred them to another specialist he had worked with to help fertility challenged couples. That specialist said he had found success in similar cases by prescribing the woman with aspirin and progesterone suppositories. There were no guarantees, but at that point, the couple was willing to try anything that could help.

As per her previous pattern, Krystin needed to put the past behind her with a major event. This time it came in the form of attending a friend's wedding in Vanuatu. They had a wonderful island holiday and fell pregnant naturally during the week that they returned home.

A bleed at five weeks was worrying, but both doctors reassured her. At 13 weeks, she stopped the progesterone and found out her baby was a girl. At 36 weeks, she stopped the aspirin and a week later, she noticed reduced foetal movement and rushed to hospital.

"It was terrifying. When the nurse pushed, the baby wasn't pushing back. The nurse was freaking out and I was beyond that. She got the doppler machine and heard the baby. She said, 'Gosh, I thought you'd lost her.' I told her I could tell from her face. It was the most horrific moment of my life."

The baby was induced the following week. After 12 hours labour, Krystin was not dilating. They infused her with oxytocin* and that worked well. She was then given an epidural, and the bag of oxytocin ran out and was replaced. All of a sudden, everything stopped. Looking back, Krystin wonders if the bag was accidentally replaced with saline instead of oxytocin.

Her doctor was in theatre and stopped by to see how she was progressing. He had expected the baby to be born. An ultrasound revealed that the baby's head was in a position where she wasn't pushing on the cervix to open it. By this time, another new bag was required and all of a sudden, everything started again. The doctor told Krystin that he was going to theatre to do another caesarean, and if the baby was not born by the time he returned, he would take her down and do a caesarean on her.

> **"I freaked out. I did not want a caesar, I just hadn't prepped myself for it. I rang my mum, crying that I have to go for a caesar, saying, 'What am I going to do? I have to take Mia to school, and I won't be able to drive.' All of those things were worrying me."**

Then the nurse checked and Krystin was fully dilated. At that moment, the doctor walked in ready to deliver so Krystin's parents, who were there with her, offered to leave the room but she asked them to stay. Three pushes later, Willow was born.

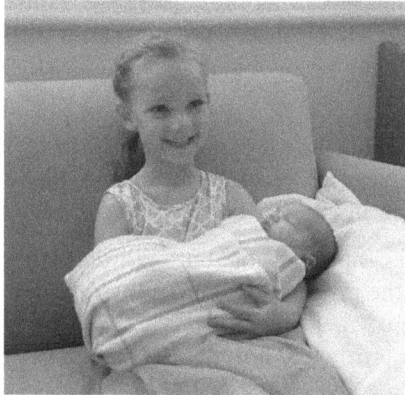

Mia meeting Willow

Krystin wanted to breastfeed, but Willow had problems latching.

> **"We fought so long to have her, so I was going to enjoy this. I decided I wasn't going to be the stressed-out mum that I was with Mia...back then I came out in a full body rash over not being about to feed. So, I asked the nurse for formula."**

I asked Krystin what she learned from her experience.

> **"I am stronger now, more aware of myself and what I need to do if I'm in this sort of situation. Obviously, Mia and Willow are the best things. Matt and I, our relationship is stronger. He's seen me at my lowest. Matt doesn't actually show that**

much emotion, but no one has ever seen me at my low as much as he has. I'll always be super appreciative of him. He's a great husband and father."

Today, Krystin's life is full—she is a busy mum of two girls, and also back at work. She now sees things differently, a little more maturely. Her life experience has given her perspective on what's really important in life.

Krystin realises that there are many women who are going through a similar journey to hers. She talks freely about her miscarriages and her friends often refer her to women who are facing the same trauma. Krystin has finally found peace and contentment and one day, hopes to contribute further in the perinatal space by becoming a midwife.

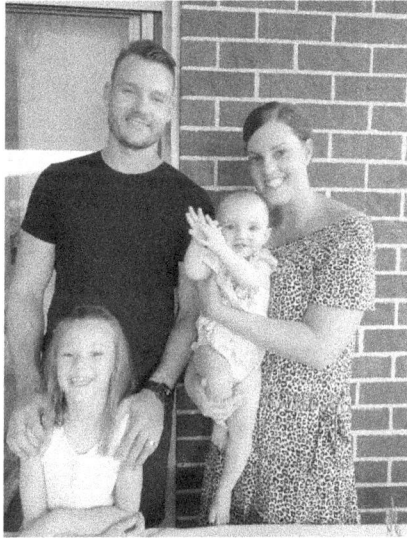

Matt, Krystin, Mia and Willow

"Everyone's different, but I like to talk about it. It makes me feel like it happened, the baby was real, I had real emotions about it. I had feelings about the babies, and for someone to come over and just sit there, and ask me about it, that helped me. That was therapy for me. It wasn't as if it never happened. It happened, I had feelings about it, it happened."

10

SARA

- Annie, aged 19
- Oliver, aged 18
- Jonathon, lived 14 hours, 2005
- Josiah, 11 years

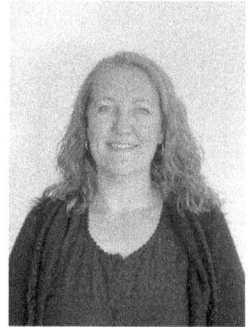

When Sara finished high school in the regional town of Warilla, her enquiring mind hungered for new experiences. She applied to attend a university in the city of Sydney and was accepted to begin a science degree. It was a huge change: making new friends, going out and enjoying the nightlife and also working a part-time job.

After her first year, Sara wasn't sure if a degree was something she wanted to continue, so she set herself a challenge. If she found a job in the two weeks before the new semester started, she would defer for a year and work full-time. That decision changed the entire course of her life—within days she started working at Microsoft, and there she met her future husband!

Sara and Dave enjoyed a whirlwind romance. Sara was only 19 when they met, 21 when they married, and 25 when she gave birth to their first child, Annie. Apart from a little nausea, Sara can't remember anything but an easy pregnancy and natural birth.

When Annie was around 11 months, Sara discovered she was pregnant again.

"My grandmother was the same, apparently all my family along the line are like that. My grandmother used to say, 'Your grandfather just had to hang up his pants and I'd be pregnant.'"

Oliver was born just 20 months after Annie. Sara contracted a virus just before going into labour, and her doctors are of the opinion that this may have stimulated labour. Sara's white blood cell count was extremely elevated, and Oliver was put on oxygen immediately after birth.

With an APGAR* score of four out of 10, Oliver was whisked away to special care.

"I couldn't hold him. That was traumatic for me at the time."

After several days, mother and baby were discharged, and Sara now had two babies under the age of two. It was a lot to handle, but Sara reflects that it was good because the two siblings would play well together.

Following Oliver, Sara decided that contraception was a good idea until they were ready for a third child. Surprisingly, when the decision was made to have a third child, it took six months for Sara to fall pregnant but when she did, she relaxed, fully expecting this pregnancy to proceed the same as her previous two.

Sara experienced a little bleeding, but her doctor assured her that it was normal. At around 10 weeks, she went to her first ultrasound and when the sonographer measured the size of the baby and discovered that she was three weeks further along than expected.

The sonographer looked more closely and told Sara that she could not see the baby's hand.

"I said, 'I don't care. The heart's beating and everything else is okay. I'm happy. Don't worry about the hand. That's all right.' I was just happy I was three weeks ahead and if there was a little deformity in the hand, we could work that out."

Dave wanted to attend the 19-week scan and because they didn't have a babysitter, the children came along as well. Trying to organise the whole family made them 15 minutes late for the appointment and the sonographer was extremely upset because it meant that the rest of her day would run late.

"She started scanning and then her demeanour changed. I could tell, and I knew something was not quite right, but I

wouldn't let myself believe it. The 13-week scan had been fine. The heart was beating. That's always the thing. The heart's beating. That's great. The brain was there. And then she started being overly nice to me. It was like she flicked a switch from angry to caring."

The sonographer left the room to get the doctor. Dave had taken the kids for an ice-cream which meant Sara was alone when the doctor went through all the things that were wrong with her baby. She recalls how horrendous it was to sit there while she was told that he had only half a brain; that his bowel was on the outside of his body, within the umbilical cord; and that he had deformed hands and feet.

"And they said, 'He's most likely not going to survive'. It was like a knife to the stomach, metaphorically speaking. I just wanted the world to swallow me up. I just felt like I wanted to get that baby out of there. I wanted to run. Often when I'm under stress I just want to hide, or run, I want to leave a job cause it's getting tough or whatever. And this was one of those times where I just went, no, I've got to get away. I can't deal with this."

With such devastating news to process, I asked Sara how she was able to communicate the information to Dave and the children waiting outside. Sara recalls walking out, seeing her kids jumping all over the place. She has the ability to shut down emotions, to go into a professional mode and tuck away her feelings because they can't be dealt with right then and there. It is her coping mechanism, and she used it that day, saying to Dave, "He's not going to survive. There are problems. We'll have to talk about it later."

They found someone to look after the kids and headed off to the Royal North Shore Hospital for a specialist scan. Sara's mother, a nurse and sonographer herself, met them there for the ultrasound.

The good news was that the baby's brain was intact. However, the new scan picked up some additional problems. He had a horseshoe shaped kidney, formed by the fusion across the midline of two distinct kidneys. The doctor also suspected Edwards Syndrome* or Trisomy 18*, a condition where he was unlikely to survive much more than a week.

To confirm the diagnosis, Sara had an amniocentesis* test. They were sent to a room to wait for the results. Doctors had already informed them of their options to terminate or carry to term. They were told that there was a 50% chance that he would be born alive, and a 10% chance he wouldn't survive the first day. They faced a decision that no parent should ever have to make.

The wait for their test results was agonising. What should they do? Amidst the turmoil, Sara noticed a small plaque on the wall. It was a verse from Psalm 139:16 that read, "Your eyes saw my unformed body; all the days ordained for me were written in your book before one of them came to be."

> **"Gosh, it was a message. It was like, it's not my choice. I know people have a choice. We were given a choice. Do we terminate now? Or do we want to wait to carry to term? And I thought, if there's just a chance. It's not my choice. I didn't want to carry that decision that I was the reason why he didn't live all the days out that were designed for him. So, we decided to carry to term."**

I asked Sara if Dave agreed and she confirmed that they were totally united in their decision. Sara recalls crying a river of tears, thankful to share her pain with their Bible Study group. Dave found it difficult to discuss and to hear Sara talk at the meetings, but despite his reticence, the emotional support and practical help that the group provided to their family was of crucial importance in helping them to get through the trauma.

One of the most difficult things that Sara dealt with during the pregnancy was the well-meaning comments of others. People would see her tummy and say things like, "Congratulations! You're having a baby! When are you due?" Or, "Oh, how exciting, a little brother or sister…"

> **"Most of the time I had to fake it. Because I didn't want to put that pain on somebody else. I didn't want to have to explain. I guess if I was a bit more unconcerned about them and more concerned about myself, I would probably have said, 'Oh, he's going to die.' But I couldn't do that."**

It became a weird balance of kindness to others and self-preservation for Sara. She is an empath and feels another person's pain deeply. Sara knew that if she told them her pain, then they too would feel it, and then she would feel the weight of two people's pain.

Explaining such a complex issue to their children proved to be another challenge. Annie and Oliver were five and three at the time, an age when they have no filter and say exactly what they think. Sara feels that they were quite oblivious during her pregnancy. They saw her tummy growing and would ask questions like, "Where will he sleep?"

"I think the thing that broke me the first time was knowing that they had to lose a brother. I could deal with it, but it wasn't fair on them."

Sara looked for resources to help her children understand, and she read a small book called 'Coping with Grief' by Mal and Dianne McKissock. It helped her realise that children don't understand death, they understand the here and now. The book suggested that they tell the kids that the baby is sick, giving them an indication of why their mum is sad and preparing them for what was to come.

Physically, the pregnancy progressed fine. He did not move as much and was smaller than her previous two babies. Sara was attending The Maternal-Fetal Medicine Centre that provides care for high-risk pregnancies. The centre has specialised staff and midwives who understand the emotional trauma these mothers are experiencing. Sara formed a bond with Kathy, a midwife who was a 'fantastic ray of sunshine.' At Sara's regular check-ups, Kathy became more than someone who physically checked on her pregnancy. She genuinely cared about Sara's wellbeing, becoming a counsellor who Sara could confided in. It was agreed between Kathy, the doctors and Sara that an induction would be best.

"Knowing the baby would be born on a predicted day was easier for me to deal with. I couldn't handle not knowing when I would go into labour – would it be at night? Would Dave be around? And we could make sure the kids were able to come and see him straight away because we didn't know how much time he had."

Two days before her due date, Sara was induced through an IV drip, early in the morning. She explained to me that because the baby had a low prognosis, the baby was not monitored. The birth process was all about focusing on her, the mother, and getting through labour in the best way possible. It was also an opportunity for new doctors to learn. The Royal North Shore is a teaching hospital, and Sara remembers having an audience of 12 people watching her give birth.

To cope with the situation, Sara had emotionally shut herself off from the world at that point. She was just going through the motions, doing what she knew she must. Through the hours and hours of labour, Sara did not know if her baby was dead or alive. When Jonathon was born alive, weighing 2.6 kg, it was an absolute miracle.

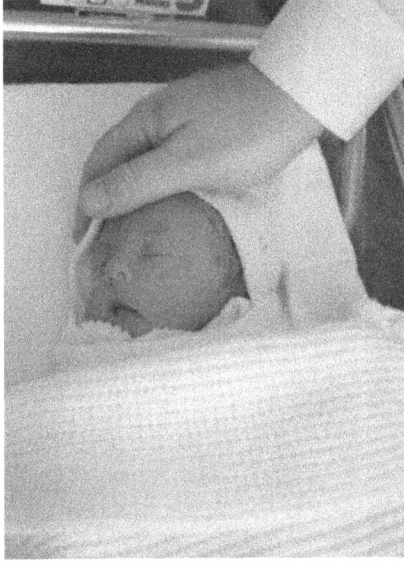

Jonathon

"It was just a surreal experience. He actually moved his head on his own. It was like, 'Oh my gosh, he's alive!' They wrapped him up and I tried to feed him. We actually dressed him. His bowel was on the outside of his body, it was all in the umbilical cord, so they had to wrap him in glad wrap to keep it tight to his body. Just so that it would be more comfortable for him. And none of the other stuff you saw. His hands were kind of quite clawed underneath and his feet were rocker bottoms, but his face was perfect, a beautiful little face."

The hospital arranged a private parent room for the family. It was set up as an actual bedroom with a double bed and curtains on the windows so that it felt more homely than a sterile medical ward. This provided a comfortable space for the family come in and visit and this is where Sara's parents brought Annie and Oliver to meet their brother.

It was an emotionally complex situation. Sara had her brave face on for her children. It felt like pretending to rejoice that Jonathon was born alive, while knowing his true prognosis.

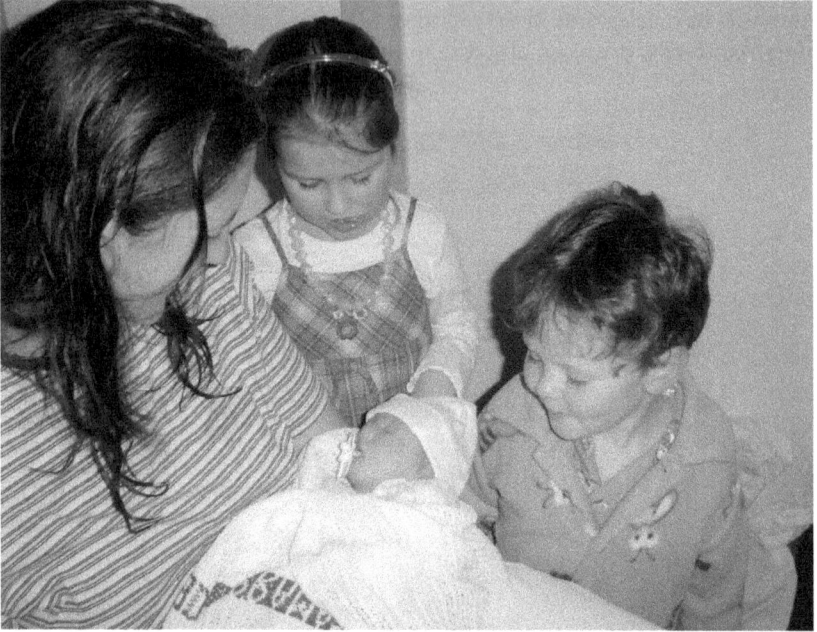

Sara, Annie and Oliver with Jonathon

"It was so emotional seeing him and all of his bits on the outside and all of that. I don't deal with that very well. It was gut-churning in some respects. And you have to try and mask it. And so, I was kind of masking all day, so by nine o'clock, we were absolutely spent."

Even though they were exhausted, neither Sara nor Dave wanted to sleep as they realised their time with Jonathon was so precious. It was during these late evening hours that they connected with the midwife on duty.

"She was the most beautiful representation of a hug I could ever, ever imagine. She sat there and talked to us. She also went to church, so she was able to connect to us on a spiritual level, and she was just amazing. She helped us get through that last little bit."

The midwife took Jonathon out of the room at midnight as he was becoming distressed. It gave Sara and Dave a chance to sleep, if only for a few hours. Around five o'clock in the morning, the nurses brought him back, saying, 'He hasn't got long." Sara and Dave put him in between them on the double bed and lay with him until he passed away.

"It was one of the most confronting things. I didn't know how people died. I'd never seen it before. They take a breath then there's nothing. Is that it? Then another breath. Is that it? You don't really know until time has passed. It was so hard."

Even though Sara had been prepared for the outcome, she was surprised by the depth of her sadness. The knot of grief hurt so badly. She needed to deal with it in her own way, a process that she likened to the nature of a cat, a creature that goes away, hides and works things out alone.

But there were practical tasks that had to be taken care of, including arrangements for Jonathon's funeral. This is where members of their church stepped in to help. They had attended the same church for over five years, and these people were their extended family. They had walked through the entire journey together and they too were grieving.

Sara spoke of the incredible kindness as people pitched in to arrange a fitting funeral to honour Jonathon. One person organised a creche to look after the children during the service, others prepared afternoon tea for all of the guests. Musicians offered to play music. It showed Sara how important it is for all those grieving to get to some point of closure and acceptance. By graciously receiving their support, it helped the family through their grieving process.

Sara's sister-in-law and her children painted a huge, white drape filled with lots of colour and rainbows. The drape covered the coffin stand and was a way to help her nephews deal with Jonathon's loss, and that of their own baby brother Thomas, who they had lost two years prior. Thomas was three months older than Oliver and he was gone suddenly with meningitis at eight weeks. That was the first time that death had touched Sara's life. She believes that her nephew's passing may have partially prepared her for what she now faced.

"You expect to see a coffin that's at least six-foot long and it's dark timber. But to see a white coffin that you can carry with two hands, it's just not right. It's not the order that you expect life to be. But also, it helped me understand what people around me were going through too. Because I was that person back then, who didn't feel like my sadness was justifiable because my sister-in-law was the one who lost the baby. But it still counts. Everybody's sadness counts."

One of Sara's favourite anecdotal stories from the day of Jonathon's funeral is something her friend experienced in a carpark close to the church. A well-dressed lady was obviously in a huff, unable to find a parking space. She saw Sara's friend and asked, "What's going on over there? I can't get a park anywhere." Sara's friend answered, "It's a funeral, actually." The lady commented, "Oh, well it must be someone really important to have this many people here." Sara's friend replied, "It was actually a 14-hour old baby." The lady's huffy attitude changed instantly.

"It was that realisation that everything is not about us. That all these circumstances, all these things we have to deal with are part of life, part of a community."

Sara and I discussed the different ways in which people show their grief. As Australians, we had both observed that we culturally deal with emotions in a rather British 'stiff upper lip' manner where we do not show our feelings, whereas other cultures, such as African, South American, Asian and European are different.

"They wail, they carry on, and they're very outward with their grief. I admire that. I find that hard. But I actually admire that because I feel like that kind of outpouring, allowing the sadness to come, allowing yourself to be sad, or whatever in that moment, helps you continue on that journey of learning acceptance."

Dave processed his grief differently to Sara.

"He started out sharing the grief with me and we cried together. So many tears! But my sadness was deeper and difficult for him to understand. I had bonded with the baby I carried, and he didn't get that chance. We just processed the grief in different ways. He grieved the loss of our connection, while I grieved the loss of Jonathon. Because we grieved so differently it kind of drove a wedge between us."

If not for their faith, Sara thinks that they would have split up. For six months there was angst, disconnection and fighting. How did she get through this period? It was her close group of friends, her own analysis and self-talk, and a continual commitment to journaling.

Sara has developed a self-talk ritual that she finds is a beneficial way to understand and work through difficult emotions.

"I do this self-talk thing all the time. I'm feeling a little bit off. What am I feeling off about? And I'll go through all the things that have happened that day. Was it this? No, was it that? No.

And then I'll think of something and bang, it'll get stronger and I'll go, Oh, that's it. Why is it bothering me? And I'll do the whole analysis thing."

She also used journaling to pour out her emotions, noticing that as she handwrote her thoughts, her brain automatically formulated understanding, creating crystallising moments of self-realisation.

The loss of Jonathon also affected Annie and Oliver. Annie was five years old and very mature for her age. Her behaviour changed dramatically from calm and cautious to moments of emotional, sometimes angry, outbursts. At the time, Sara didn't understand what was happening, but now she kicks herself because she has since learned the value of just being there.

"I was so busy dealing with my own grief that I couldn't see rationally outside of that to say she needs help, she needs someone. I did take her to the school counsellor, but at the time I remember just feeling bewildered. How do I help my little girl? She was drawing in black and had stopped drawing in colour. She would scream back at me and she'd never done that her whole life. We now know that she's autistic, but at the time I didn't know that."

Sara thought about how she could get some positivity back into Annie's life, and started to draw a happy place. She invited Annie to help, doing the drawing so her daughter could just talk. They drew a river, and mountains, trees and a picnic with lots of colour. She put that on the wall to help Annie reframe her thoughts.

Both children were soaking up the feelings of their parents—they saw mum crying and sensed the emotional tension between their parents. In Annie, this emerged as anxiety, but Oliver, who was only three at the time, had a much more childlike and simplistic view of the situation. He assessed things from his day-to-day experiences, asking, "Mum, who's going to feed Jonathon in heaven?"

Slowly, Sara moved to what she calls a "coping place", her name for the state where she could function but didn't feel whole. There was still a part of her that wasn't right. Little things would trigger her like Huggies nappies commercials, hearing babies cry, or milestone dates. One of their closest friends had a baby boy five days after Jonathon, and he was a constant reminder.

"In the beginning, it was really difficult. But they are our dearest friends and they made us godparents. It became part of the healing process to have someone to love and buy gifts for."

As time went on, the couple were undecided about whether or not to conceive again. They had been told that there was a slight increase in the possibility of having another baby with chromosomal abnormalities. The sad thing was that they actually knew a woman who had two consecutive babies with chromosomal abnormalities, and it was devastating.

"I was thinking, what if we're that too? You know, I don't get to say that we get another healthy baby. I needed someone to say to me that it's going to be fine. It will be great. But Dave didn't want that either. He didn't want more stress on our marriage. So, we decided, nope, that's it. Get rid of all the baby stuff."

A couple of years later, they decided to look for a new home closer to Dave's place of work and the children's new school. They found the right house and signed the contracts, only to discover they were pregnant!

For Sara, the anxiety at each scan was horrendous. By the 19-week scan, she was a mess. Even though she could rationalise her way through her thoughts, Sara went in with her heart racing. She was completely on edge, attending on her own because Dave was working, and the children were at school. One blessing was that she returned to the high-risk maternity unit and the same wonderful midwife was there to care for her.

"Even though everything was fine, I suddenly realised, I can't replace that baby. There was some healing in having another baby that was healthy. But Jonathon was still dead, there was that finality. I can't take that away. I can't reduce that in any way and that will stay.

So, I think once that point happened, I was able to enjoy each day, but I didn't buy baby furniture until the 11th hour. I could never, never rest in that expectation that this baby was going to come home and spend the rest of his life with us."

Dave was over the moon with excitement at the new pregnancy. Everything went as smoothly as with her other three pregnancies, and at 39 weeks, they made the decision to induce. Just as they were leaving for the hospital, Sara noticed that Annie was upset. She was anxious and panicked and Sara could see how much Jonathon's loss had affected her.

Sara remembered a little opal necklace that Dave had bought as a spare gift and thought it would be perfect to help Annie. Sara told her that the opal came out of the ground, it had been there a long time, God had put it there and made it beautiful. So, God would look after them too. Sara feels that it gave her something tangible to hold onto.

On Valentine's day 2008, Josiah entered the world, a healthy boy. Sara noticed the immediate difference in Annie—his birth was healing for her as well. Oliver was ecstatic and asked, "Can we keep this one?"

Josiah is now 11 years old and Annie and Oliver are at the end of their schooling years. Sara has been a working mother with positions in administration while raising her three children, all of whom are diagnosed with autism spectrum disorder*.

"With all the stuff we've had to deal with, I'm like, too much. This is not right. This is too much for one lifetime. Enough."

Sara has courageously supported her children and, in the past few years, she realised that at 44, she has yet to fulfil her own potential. She is currently studying psychology at university and hopes to use her talents and knowledge to make a difference to others.

"It's a slow process, emotions, learning and growing from experiences rather than letting them spiral out of control. Some people can't, they need help to be able to do that. I'm just hoping that people will have more awareness and acceptance of different ways of grieving and processing and learning about emotions to be able to make their lives better from it."

11

YVETTE

- Anorexia Bulimia*
- CIN3*
- Three Miscarriages
- Pre-eclampsia
- Rainbow baby: Dimitri, aged eight
- Polycystic Ovary Syndrome (PCOS)
- Postnatal Depression (PND)

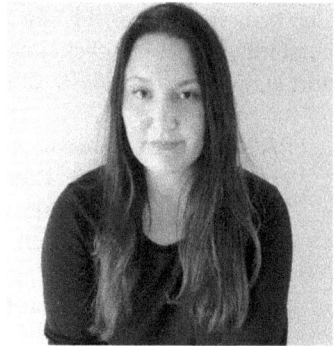

B oy meets girl next door. They fall in love. It sounds like a cliché, but that's exactly how Yvette and Steve met. Yvette was 21, studying for her Bachelor of Arts degree exams on a Saturday night. She heard a fight going on outside, opened her window to find out what was happening and saw a man sitting on the rooftop next door, eating a chocolate bar. That was her introduction to the man who would be her husband.

The couple started dating, and within six months, Yvette discovered she was pregnant. It was a completely unplanned shock for the couple, but they loved each other and wanted to keep the baby. They immediately made plans for accommodating their new addition, discussing changes including deferring university and buying a house together.

Yvette went in for her first scan. All she could see was an empty sac, but her doctor reassured her that it was still early days. He suggested that she return for another scan in two weeks. Happy with the explanation, Yvette went home and noticed that she was bleeding. She phoned Steve and told him what was happening, and the two went straight into the Royal Price Alfred Hospital Emergency Department where she was ushered straight through.

After examining her, the doctor was quite optimistic. He explained that Yvette's cervix was still closed, so the baby could be fine. She stayed in hospital overnight, and though she continued to bleed, the staff advised that bleeding in early pregnancy is normal. Yvette was discharged and went home.

> **"I went to the bathroom and I knew I miscarried. I saw it and I was just so distraught. I just remember sleeping the whole day. And I remember my husband ringing up my family, saying, 'Look, I'm just ringing to let you know that Yvette was pregnant, but she miscarried.'"**

Steve and Yvette had felt quite differently about the miscarriage. Steve is seven years older than Yvette, and he was ready to start a family. He was quite emotional about the loss. For Yvette, there were mixed emotions.

> **"Why did it happen to me? That baby would have been dead when I was at the scan. My doctor was very comforting. He said, 'Look, it's common.' Some people get offended because my family would say, 'Don't worry, you're still young,' and that didn't offend me, it actually gave me comfort."**

Yvette mentally rationalised all of the reasons why it was probably better this way. She was only 22 and she was not actively trying for a baby. There was no need to rush into buying a house and now she could complete her studies. Despite the logic of her thinking, Yvette remembers the whole experience as being physically draining, and the pregnancy hormones in her body made her emotional state see-saw up and down. She started her second year of university feeling anxious.

> **"I got amazing support from my university. I actually went to one of the university pastors. He's one of the lecturers in counselling and psychology and because I was Catholic at the time, they actually did the healing of the sick for me because there's a church on the campus. That really helped a lot, having the right support."**

Later that year, Yvette's girlfriend had a baby and she was happy to tell me that she felt no resentment, but only excitement and happiness for her friend. It was a beautiful distraction and she attended the baby shower with the intention of being present and enjoying the moment. Yvette has lots of cousins and friends with children and she is grateful that she has never found time with them to be triggers for sadness.

On their first anniversary, Yvette and Steve went to Bali for a holiday, and shortly after, moved in together. A few years later, Steve proposed, and the couple married.

In 2012, Yvette fell pregnant. Though unplanned, they were happy to start their family. Yvette had difficulties from early on, experiencing spotting and cramping. Instead of morning sickness, she had all-day sickness—for the first six months she lived on crackers and water!

> **"I was very, very nervous during the first three months. I would wake up every morning and go to the toilet, thinking, 'Is today the day I will miscarry?' Then we went to get scanned and they asked me, 'How many weeks do you think you are?' I said, 'Five or six.' They said, 'You're almost nine weeks and there's his heartbeat.' I was so relieved, A lot of my burdens just went, vanished."**

At 24 weeks gestation, Yvette was diagnosed with pre-eclampsia. This caused her to retain fluid, and she remembers her puffy face and extremities, describing her feet as "So swollen they looked like dinosaur feet!" This was especially difficult as she was working full-time in retail, on her feet all day.

Yvette stopped working at 36 weeks and was looking forward to a month of rest before motherhood. The baby's due date was coincidentally the same day that she had miscarried four years earlier. Yvette remarked that this was freaky, but she knew that this time, things would be different.

The doctor prescribed bedrest for the last four weeks of Yvette's pregnancy. She was already experiencing Braxton Hicks* contractions, and in her 37th week, the contractions intensified dramatically signalling active labour.

Steve whisked Yvette into hospital, and she was given gas* as pain relief. Her waters would not break, so she was given a morphine shot. The pain worsened and Yvette asked for an epidural but it was too late—Dimitri was born after just six hours of labour, weighing 3.3kg.

> **"He was perfect, a healthy little chubba. I didn't need stitches. The doctor said, 'It looks like you didn't have a baby, you're so lucky.' I couldn't believe it!"**

Yvette chose to breastfeed Dimitri, and at one point, he kept crying during feeding. She contacted the Australian Breastfeeding Association and asked for help.

"I told them he was not taking the milk. They asked, 'How much are you pumping?' I said, '350 mils.' They said, 'That's good for both boobs.' I'm like, 'No, that's for one boob.' So, I found out I had too much milk. I had to pump a little bit then feed him, then pump again. It was exhausting."

Dimitri was then diagnosed with reflux and colic. Yvette had to avoid any foods that affected him because it was being passed through her breast milk. Her bra cup size had increased from a C to an E, and she described herself to me as a stick with big boobs!

The reflux and colic also upset Dimitri's sleep. He cried constantly, wanting to be held upright. Yvette had returned to part-time work after five months, and then to full-time work after nine months. She was still breastfeeding morning and night and expressing throughout the day. The first-time parents were beyond fatigued.

Looking back, Yvette wishes she had taken two years maternity leave. She compared herself to other new mothers who seemed to be coping easily. Furthermore, her immigrant grandparents had arrived in a new country, continued to work and have babies, as did her in-laws, so she thought that it must be like this for everyone.

"I was young, 27 at the time and if other people could do it, we could do it. My husband thought I had a problem, but I denied it. He was just as exhausted as me because we were sharing the load of looking after him and we were just fried by the time the weekend came. It was madness."

It took a massive fight with Steve to get Yvette to the doctor. She was diagnosed with PND, and prescribed anti-depressants, with referrals to a psychologist and a psychiatrist.

"I probably drove him nuts because I didn't want to talk. We all have our masks. One day Steve and I had another massive fight and he said, 'That's it. I'm going to take Dimitri and I'm going to get full custody of everything. I can't take this anymore.' And then I wanted to kill myself. I was on my way to do it, but my husband wouldn't stop calling me. I finally answered and said, 'You need to take me to ED (Emergency Department).'"

Steve took her to the ED where Yvette saw a psychiatrist and told him everything. He assessed her mental health and recommended that she voluntarily admit herself to the psychiatric ward.

> **"It was such a surreal experience, like the mental institutions you see in the movies. I met with another psychiatrist and they couldn't get through to me. I was sitting there, saying, 'I just want to take my life.' They said, 'But what about your son? Don't you want to be there for him and live?' I said, 'No, he's better off without me.'"**

She was put in the acute ward overnight with two other women who were unstable and one of them needed to be sedated. Yvette recalls thinking that she was going to die there. In that moment, she didn't want to die and instead lay in bed awake all night.

Thankfully, they moved her to a calmer ward the following day. Due to her heightened state, the doctors increased her anti-depressant medication and started her on sleeping tablets and Valium to combat her anxiety. But this where Yvette's healing began.

> **"I really hit rock bottom. When I look back, I feel like I'm talking about another person. I've gone through anorexia bulimia. I was very body obsessed when I was a teenager, then I had an abusive partner, which led me to getting CIN3*. Even though that was so stressful, I never went through depression back then and I never thought about taking my life."**

Hospitalisation gave Yvette the chance to take time out. She began to write ferociously, trying to process her emotions and to heal her mind. This took a huge toll on her relationship with Steve, who said that normally, people go to the hospital to visit someone who has had a baby, or someone who is sick. But for him, he felt that there was nothing worse than going to hospital to visit his wife in the psychiatric unit.

After a few weeks, she felt well enough to leave, but this too was difficult. Steve and Yvette agreed to a separation that lasted for around two months. They were brought back together because the tenants moved out from the property they had purchased as their family home. They moved to the new home together and began the hard task of rebuilding their relationship. Yvette described it as "baby steps, a lot of one step forward and one step back."

Yvette recently looked back at photos of herself at that time and noticed how sad she looked with her hollow eyes and sunken face. She had many demons and was trying to find her way forward.

"I was just trying to find a sense of normal again and that was really hard because I was still in denial of my illness, but I knew there was something wrong with me."

It was another accidental pregnancy that ended in early miscarriage that tipped Yvette back over the edge. A short time after this, she tried to take her life with an overdose of sleeping pills.

"All I remember is waking up and then here I am at St. George hospital. And they wanted to put me into psychiatric care. I begged, 'No please don't, just don't. I don't want to go back there.' So, instead Steve put me into a yoga retreat."

This three-day retreat was pivotal to Yvette's recovery. She made the effort to attend every class. She practiced mindfulness and yoga. She read books on yoga and philosophy, went to a naturopathy consultation and had a massage. She returned feeling so much better, even her psychologist was pleased with her mental state.

Yvette weaned herself off all her medications. She continued to eat well, to practice yoga and most importantly, took time out for herself. She was doing very well until another unplanned pregnancy in 2017.

"I felt so sick with this pregnancy, to the point where Dimitri touched me and said, 'Mum, you're boiling.' I remember going to the bathroom and it happened. But I felt really broken because I thought, yeah, we can have a kid now because I'm past the PND and I'm in such a good place. It would have been the perfect time to have a baby."

After this third miscarriage, Yvette searched for answers. A few years before, she had been diagnosed with PCOS and her doctor informed her that this was the likely cause of her miscarriages.

"I felt really, really broken. I could feel that cloud and I fell into PND again."

The doctor's diagnosis was factual, but it was devastating to Yvette in her fragile emotional and mental state. She sought out help from the priest at her son's school, seeking spiritual guidance and for someone to listen without judgement while she poured out her feelings freely.

The talk was very helpful, and it encouraged Yvette be transparent with Steve. It has helped the couple to communicate better and to plan for a future together.

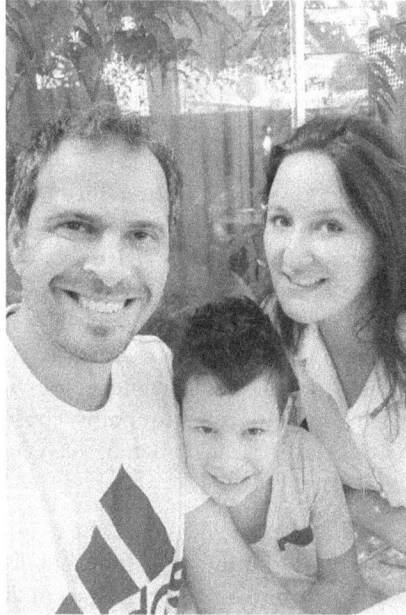

Steve, Dimitri and Yvette

"They asked if we wanted to do IVF, but I said no. It was a personal decision that I just didn't want to go through it. It's a really heartbreaking process and I already do have one child.

We've decided that's it, no more unplanned pregnancies. I just really love being a family of three, and even though I'm probably the only mum in my son's year that has only one child, it doesn't matter because that little boy is enjoying life so much and so am I."

Yvette continues to work on herself every day. Some days are more difficult than others, but she keeps moving forward.

Yvette is using her personal experience and professional skills to connect with and encourage others who are experiencing life challenges. Her Facebook page, 'She is Sacred' has a following of more than 12,000.

Started in 2015 to document her PND, her mental health, her marriage and womanhood, Yvette has had both men and women reach out to her to tell their stories.

> **"It's been cathartic for me, and it takes a little bit of their pain for a brief moment which is really nice. I think it is really heartbreaking how miscarriage has affected people After I posted the poem I wrote a couple of months ago, I've had people commenting saying, I miscarried 30, 40, 50 years ago and that pain still doesn't go away, that grief, that longing. I am really lucky to have my boy, he's a miracle."**

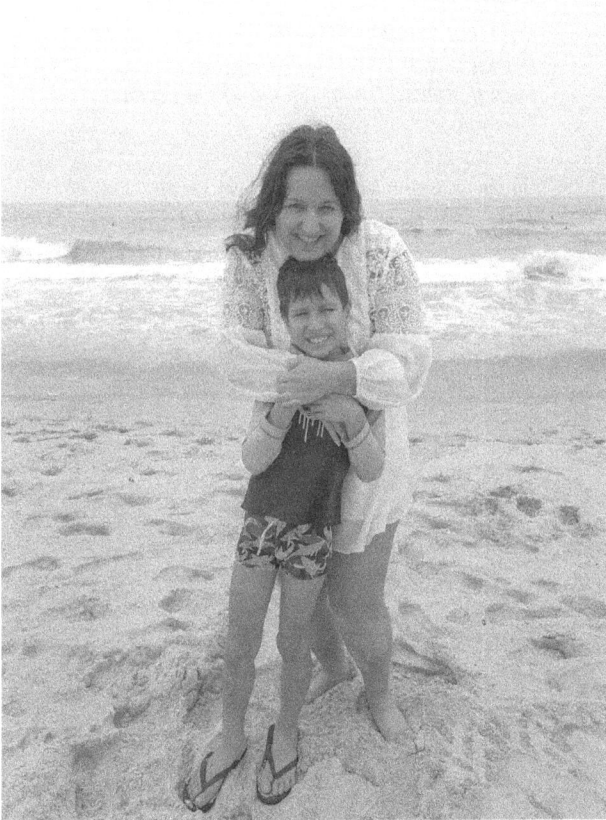

Yvette and Dimitri

To the woman who is grieving over her loss.
Even if it is her first loss, or multiple loss.
Even if it is a missed miscarriage.
Even if it is an ectopic pregnancy.
Even if it is a failed IVF round.
I see you.

To the woman who is grieving over her loss.
Even if it is an early miscarriage.
Even if she did not know the sex.
Even if the scan could not find a heartbeat.
Even if it is an empty sac.
I see you.

To the woman who is grieving over her loss.
Even if it was past 20 weeks.
Even if it was born sleeping.
Even if it passed away days, weeks or months
I see you.

To the woman who is grieving over her loss.
Even if she has not been able to start a family yet.
Even if she has a child.
Even if she has more than one child.
I see you.

To the woman who is grieving over her loss.
She is broken.
She is empty.
She is confused.
I see you.

To the woman who is grieving over her loss.
I see you.

— **YVETTE MYSTAKAS, SHE IS SACRED**

12

RENEE

- Zac, aged 12, Meconium Aspiration Syndrome (MAS)*, Reflux and Pneumonia
- Jake, aged 10, Silent Reflux*, Sever's Disease*

R enee is the daughter of my close friends, a couple I have considered family for almost 20 years. We have shared and supported each other through the many ups and downs of life. Renee's story is one that needs to be heard and so I asked her and her parents, Tony and Dianne, to share their memories for this book.

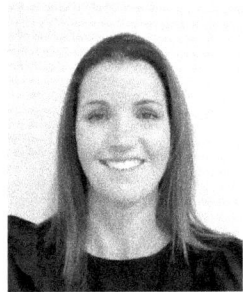

It started with the chance meeting on a big night out. Tim comes from a small country town in Southern NSW, while Renee grew up in Wollongong, about an hour's drive south of Sydney. They had both moved to the city for work and a livelier social life that had not been available in their hometowns.

Tim and Renee started out as friends and over the course of the following years, they dated. It was seven years on when they decided to get married and start their family. Renee consulted her doctor about stopping her contraception and was warned that it could take up to a year to fall pregnant.

Contrary to predictions, it happened immediately! The wedding was scheduled for January 2007 and right before her big day, Renee discovered she was pregnant!

Their first ultrasound was at 12 weeks' gestation and included the nuchal translucency scan. Everything seemed normal except that their baby had a thicker nuchal fold, an indicator of possible Down Syndrome or other chromosomal abnormalities.

> **"It was a shock and I didn't really understand the whole thing because it was our first pregnancy. The doctor was talking about terminating. We walked out thinking, 'Did that just happen? For real?'"**

The couple was shocked that the doctor was giving them termination advice based on that one test. They were advised that a further test, an amniocentesis could be done, but that because it was an invasive test, it was risky. Tim and Renee made the decision to go ahead with the procedure and then faced the distressing waiting period when they discussed the possible outcomes.

> **"We decided, no, that's [termination] not happening. Whatever is meant to be is meant to be."**

The test results came back as normal and they were relieved to know that their baby was healthy. However, they couldn't help but feel upset that the doctor had put them through so much angst for nothing.

Renee handled pregnancy well with just a little nausea in the afternoons. She attended her regular visits with the midwife, increasing to weekly visits as full-term approached. On her actual due date, the baby was still happy and snug in her womb with no signs of being ready for birth.

The midwife checked mother and baby, and all seemed well. The doctor informed Renee that because everything seemed fine, they would not intervene until 10 days beyond the due date. If labour had not started by then, they would induce.

Each day passed with no change. Day 10 arrived and finally they went to the hospital.

> **"I went in with my suitcase, going to have a baby. I didn't have a birthing plan. I didn't go to antenatal classes. Some people say, 'I'm going to do this and I'm going to do that.' But I didn't. It's better to be flexible, I think."**

At the time, Renee had no idea how important her attitude would be over the coming days.

She was admitted on a Tuesday morning and the doctor applied gel to induce her labour.

The couple waited expectantly for something to happen, and they were soon joined by both sets of their parents who travelled up to the hospital, eager and excited to meet their first grandchild.

After 24 hours, still nothing had happened. The doctor decided to reapply the gel in the hope that the second application would do the trick. All of Wednesday passed without advancement. After two days of waiting with excited anticipation at the hospital, the couple and expectant grand parents were worn out.

Around Thursday lunchtime, Renee felt sick and vomited. It was her first contraction. The midwives told her she was going into labour.

"It was the feeling of being sick, not pain. I just felt sick with a cramping kind of pain, not intense pain."

Her waters had not broken, and she was not dilating, but at least something had started. The birthing suite had a shower and bathtub, so Renee decided to try immersion in hot water to see if it soothed the nausea and pain. She eased herself into the bath and it worked wonders until the water went cold. She got out and went straight into a hot shower to maintain the heat on her body while the bath was refilled.

"At the time, there were really severe water restrictions. We were joking, 'We're going to empty the dam for me to have this baby!' But I pretty much vomited on every contraction and the only thing that made me feel comfortable was being in water."

Thursday turned into Friday and it was now four days since she had arrived at the hospital. Renee's waters were broken by the doctor, but even that did not move things along. She was only four centimetres dilated but the pain was getting progressively worse. It had gone on for so long that Renee was physically and emotionally spent.

Realising her state, the doctor prescribed an epidural. Renee recalls the two doctors who came in to administer the injection. One was an older man, and the other appeared to be quite young. It sticks in her mind because she expected the younger man to be the trainee and other older man to be experienced, but it turned out to be the other way around. They asked for permission to allow the trainee to do the injection and Renee agreed, desperate for pain relief. Once done, the doctor suggested she should get some rest as she would likely have a few more hours of labour.

Seeing his wife settled, Tim left the room for a break while Dianne stayed with her daughter. The epidural was not working and Renee was experiencing intense pain.

> **"When Tim came back in, I was screaming that the epidural hadn't worked. So, they had to do it again. They kept coming in and checking but there was nothing, no movement and no dilating."**

That the situation had gone on for four days was beyond belief. Thinking back, Renee believes that because nothing dramatic was happening, and also because she was not the type of people to speak up and complain, she was relegated to the staff's 'check and monitor' category. Being their first baby, the couple had no idea of what to expect or what should happen, or what they should ask for—they had no measure of an acceptable level of care.

> **"I think they just left me because I didn't make enough noise to get the help that we probably needed. We were just managing it I suppose, thinking that what was happening was the way it was. I didn't know what I was doing."**

The other issue was that during the week that Renee was admitted, the birthing suite conducted 13 unplanned c-sections. These births were planned as vaginal births but were escalated to caesareans during the birth process. This put enormous strain on theatre resources and staff.

Eventually, Dianne could no longer stand to see her daughter in so much pain. She found a doctor and said to him, "She can't go on like this." It was decided that Renee should deliver by c-section and they prepped her to go straight into theatre.

Tim put on a gown and the couple went to theatre to finally deliver their baby. Out came Zac, at a whopping 4.4kg. He cried, a great sign, and his parents were told that he was healthy, but that they needed to take him to neonatal care for oxygen.

> **"I relaxed. Our parents went home because they hadn't slept for four days and as far as we knew, everything was fine. They were just going to monitor him for a bit."**

Renee settled into her room to get some well-deserved rest. The couple's parents went back to a nearby apartment they had arranged so that they could be close by for support. As soon as Renee was asleep, Tim went back to the same apartment and crashed on the couch.

At 3am, an agitated nurse came into Renee's room and woke her, saying that something was wrong and that they could not get hold of Tim. She called Tim and he wasn't answering, so she called her mum. Dianne answered the phone, half asleep, and heard Renee say that Tim needed to come back. Throwing some clothes on, Dianne roused the household and they all rushed back to the hospital.

When they arrived, Zac was surrounded by the Newborn Paediatric Emergency Transport Service (NETS)* team and their paediatrician. Fortunately, the doctor on duty had noticed that the newborn was not breathing properly and he immediately ordered an x-ray to determine the cause. That x-ray revealed that Zac had severe meconium aspiration syndrome (MAS). His lungs looked like they were painted white because he had inhaled so much meconium that they were completely coated.

The NETS team stabilised Zac and transferred him to the Royal Women's Hospital where there was a NICU equipped with staff and facilities to cope with his severe prognosis. Tim and all the other family members jumped in the car to follow the ambulance.

Dianne stayed back with Renee who was told that she was not well enough to be transported.

"They said that I could go once I was up and about, so I got up pretty quick!"

As soon as possible the next day, Renee was transferred by ambulance to be with her baby.

The families reunited in the foyer of the hospital and Renee and Tim were whisked away to NICU.

The rest of the family was distraught, not knowing what they could do to help. One of the hospital staff members saw how lost they looked and ushered them into the chapel to wait for news.

Renee stayed in the NICU for as long as she could and was grateful that the hospital also admitted her as a patient so that she could continue her own recovery while being close to her baby.

"He was put on a high frequency ventilator that was pretty much breathing for him. He went on that straight away."

Zac could not breathe on his own and could not be moved or held because of the machines and all of the tubes performing his bodily functions. He was placed in level three of the NICU, the high intensity area where he received one-on-one care from an exclusively assigned medical professional.

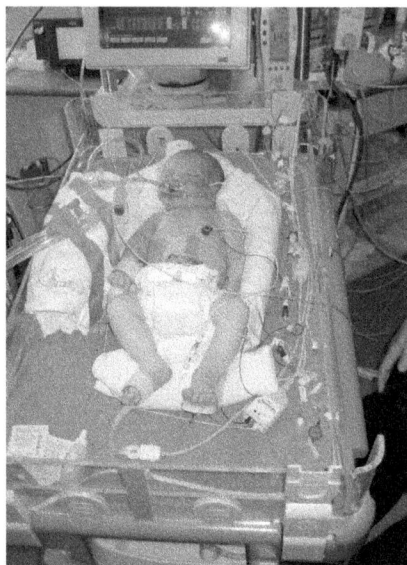

Zac in NICU

The meconium could not be extracted from Zac's lungs, so his survival was dependant on his own body's ability to break down and process the fluid. Days passed and after one week, Renee was discharged. The couple and their families stayed at the hospital every day for as long as permitted, but with the restriction that only two people were allowed in the NICU at one time, the other members of the family had to wait outside in another room, taking turns to go in and see the newborn.

Renee's milk came in and she was encouraged to express so they could give Zac the benefit of the antibodies. She would joke to her family that she was off to "milk the cows" on her way to a special room for mothers of NICU babies to express their milk. This became a kind of therapy session for all the mums, giving them the space and time to chat as they expressed.

"Talking to those people was more helpful than anything. I think the best thing was being with other people going through traumatic times. Everyone had a different story. One had

triplets who weren't full term, so she just had to be in there until they got to the spot where they could go home. And there were other people from country areas, like this one lady who had flown in and she had chicken pox, so she couldn't go and see her baby. Her husband was back on the farm and couldn't leave so she was on her own."

On one particular day when Dianne was waiting for her turn to see her grandson, she went off to a nearby shopping mall. Wandering around aimlessly, she came across a crystal shop. For some reason, she felt compelled to go inside. The shop assistant said her usual, "Hello, how are you?" and Dianne could not hold back her tears. She told the story of her grandson, and the shop assistant was so moved that she quickly gathered some crystals and holy water and gave them to Dianne as a gift for Zac.

At that point, Dianne was willing to try anything. She took the gifts back to the hospital and placed them near Zac's tiny feet, hoping they would somehow make a difference.

Anticipating that the fluid had cleared enough for his lungs to function, the doctors took Zac off the ventilator, but he still could not breathe on his own, so they had to put him straight back onto the machine. They tried again periodically without success.

Renee described those days, that stretched into weeks, as a sort of 'Groundhog Day" where they repeated the daily routine of getting up early, going to the hospital, hoping for good news, hearing that there was no change, waiting by Zac's cot all day and staying until they were told to go home.

I asked Renee how she got through this incredibly difficult time.

"I think we got through it because we've got good support and we had each other. Tim had just started his business so that just went out the window. He didn't work. We had mum and dad and everyone around. We just took one day at a time."

Renee's parents saw it as their role to support their daughter's family in any way that they could. Dianne and Tony have their own business, but they were so emotionally wrung out that they could not even think about work. They are grateful for the wonderful staff who took care of things and also their understanding clients who cooked meals and dropped in baby gifts to show their support in practical ways. Tony also assisted by providing status updates to concerned extended family and friends.

"It was good because we didn't have to tell everyone blow by blow what was happening. I had a friend that did the same. So, it was just telling those two key people rather than having to send 50 messages to everyone."

Renee spoke about the generosity of people, helping with their time, understanding and acts of kindness. This extended to Tim's clients—he had only recently started his own business, yet his clients were totally understanding of the need to put family first.

After two-and-a-half weeks of anxious waiting and watching, both the medical staff and Zac's family were becoming increasingly concerned at his lack of progress.

"The doctors said they had never seen a case as bad as his where he needed to be on a ventilator for so long. They started to think that something else was wrong."

Zac's doctor suggested that they do a lung biopsy to investigate the situation further, but the logistics of performing surgery on the newborn were complicated—it would require moving him to theatre and because of his life-support equipment, this could not easily be done. Contemplating surgery on the baby took the family's concern and worry to an even higher level.

Calling on all the resources available, Zac's doctor asked for the opinion of a paediatrician from the UK who had just joined the hospital staff. This doctor examined the newborn and told them that he had seen a similar case once before. From his experience, he recommended keeping Zac on the ventilator for a few more days. He felt that with a little more time to process the fluid, his lungs would be clear enough to function.

Sure enough, by the end of three weeks, the doctors were able to disconnect the ventilator and Zac started to breathe on his own. He was downgraded to level two in the NICU and continued to improve enough to be transferred to a hospital closer to Renee and Tim's home.

It was at this point, four weeks on from his birth, that Zac's parents were finally able to hold him for the first time, an experience that was simultaneously wonderful and awkward as they learnt how hold and feed their new bub.

"Breastfeeding took a while to get the hang of for both of us. He wasn't putting on weight and that's when we had to top-up. But the good thing was that he got some breastmilk and I think it made a big difference in helping him recover."

Renee tried using a variety of baby formulas for top-up feeding, but Zac suffered from reflux and none of the different brands seemed to agree with him. After a few months of struggling to find a solution, Renee was finally able to access a prescription-only baby formula that he was able to digest.

Zac continued on oxygen for two more weeks with the medical staff preferring that he reach 98% oxygen saturation levels before discharge. His levels plateaued at around 80% for several days but finally, six weeks on from his birth, Zac was able to go home with his mum and dad.

"I remember Tim picking me up from hospital with a new apprentice in the car. He dropped me home and then went to work. I'm like, 'What do I do now?'"

A new mum's first days with a healthy baby are challenging enough, but Renee's early motherhood had the added stress of contending with serious medical protocols. Zac had been treated with a number of drugs while in hospital and Renee had to continue with two of them at home—Viagra to support his lung function and morphine which had been used to alleviate pain and relax Zac's body while on the ventilator.

"The paediatrician said, 'Here are the scripts. You need to go to a compounding pharmacist. Go to this one that knows me because they're going to think you're a drug addict.'"

The morphine was tricky because Zac had to be weaned off it gradually. He had been taking the drug for so long that he was dependent and even though it was only a millilitre, he had to be weaned off it in tiny increments, a process that took around two months.

With all the trauma surrounding his birth, it is not surprising that Zac was unsettled. He would cry all the time and getting him to sleep, at times, felt impossible. He never slept for more than 40 minutes during the day, and woke frequently throughout the night, often waking every couple of hours.

"We tried everything. We'd go out and have this crying baby, taking turns pushing him in the pram. And people would say, 'Oh, just take him around in the car.' And I'm like, 'Don't you think I've tried that? I've tried all the tricks and it's not working.' I was an emotional wreck because it was so draining. Tim would go out in a snow jacket in the middle of the night, walking the streets with this screaming baby. Tim was exhausted, but he would come home and bath Zac every night, even when he was tired from work."

Renee felt as if she couldn't go anywhere with her newborn. She would attempt a shopping trip and he would cry in the car. When Zac was four months old, the family went on a long drive and he cried so much that Tim and Renee were at breaking point. They decided to turn his seat around so that he was facing forward and that helped immensely. They later discovered that reflux babies feel uncomfortable travelling backwards.

By the time he reached the age of one, Zac was given a clean bill of health from the Children's Hospital. He was still unsettled and wakeful throughout the night until he was around two years old, behaviour that Renee attributes to his difficult start in life.

In seeking solutions, Renee found an excellent naturopath. Her best friend had found him to be very good, so she decided to take Zac for a consultation. Her baby was diagnosed as lactose intolerant, something she wished she had known before trying all the different baby formulas. The naturopath prescribed some homeopathic remedies to help repair his body and Renee was pleased with Zac's improvement.

When he was 11 months old, the unexpected happened again—Renee realised she was pregnant! The discovery was a mixture of joy and trepidation as a result of her first birth, but this time, armed with knowledge and experience, the couple put in place a plan to ensure a smoother outcome for their second child.

Zac was born through the public health system because Tim and Renee had not upgraded their health insurance in time to cover pregnancy. By the time of the second pregnancy, everything was in place and they were able to choose a private obstetrician who would be completely responsible for their care. Renee does not blame the public hospital for Zac's condition, though she wonders what would have happened if they had performed the c-section earlier. Could he still have been born with MAS? Yes, it is possible, but perhaps it might have been less severe. Either way, with the care of their own obstetrician, the couple felt that they would have more control over the way their baby would be delivered.

With her second pregnancy, Renee had all-day nausea. The couple decided to go for their first ultrasound to confirm that all was well, but after that they chose not to do the Nuchal Translucency scan or any other scans in order to avoid the situation they had been confronted with last time.

"Tim was very strong. We both thought that if there was something wrong, then that was what we were meant to have. We weren't going to intervene. So, we didn't do any more scans."

Renee booked into a different hospital and made sure her obstetrician was aware of her past experience. She did not want to go into labour and chose to have an elective c-section. The doctor agreed.

Jake was born at a healthy weight of 3.8kg via a textbook epidural caesarean birth. It was a completely different delivery from her first with Renee home after one week. She is so thankful that Dianne came to stay during her first three weeks at home so that she could concentrate on Jake while her mum took care of 20-month-old Zac.

Breastfeeding Jake was a real challenge. Even with the help of a breast care nurse, it was difficult.

"Jake was so hungry, and I couldn't relax because it hurt. In the end, I just thought, 'You know what, it's too hard.'"

Unsure of what to do, Renee took Jake to the paediatrician who recognised the signs of silent reflux. The newborn was prescribed the same prescription formula as Zac and with the change of diet, he soon began to thrive.

After three weeks, Dianne had to return to work and Renee found herself alone with a toddler and a newborn. Neither would settle or sleep and Renee was stretched thin, struggling to manage. It got to the point where she realised that she needed help, so she called Whispers Cottage, a service that helps new mothers set a regular sleep routine for their babies.

"One day I was sitting on my bed, crying like a baby. I rang up and spoke to the lady saying, 'I've got these two crying babies. I can't do this.' She booked me in for the following Friday and it cost $400, the best $400 I've ever spent. It was just me and Jake and they gave us a routine."

Renee explained that she was given information on the best routine sleep and play times for babies at each age range. She learnt how to settle her children, and now knew what patterns she was trying to create for her sons.

"I could put him to bed awake. I wasn't sitting there rocking him, feeling like I couldn't move until he was asleep. It was just gold—my mum, my dad, anyone could do it and it didn't have to be me."

Both children have grown into active and healthy boys. Renee was warned that Zac may have learning difficulties due to his oxygen deprivation, but that has not been the case. He is active in sport and doing well at school, achieving various awards in both. Renee has noticed that whenever Zac gets sick, it is usually something to do with his respiratory system. When he was aged one and again when he was in the lower primary grades, he was diagnosed with pneumonia.

> **"He was coughing. They would say it was asthma, but I knew it wasn't, he just had a weakness in his lungs. The doctor wouldn't do anything, so I started reading up about salt therapy. I told mum and dad about it and they said one had opened up across the road from their office. We went straight there. He was struggling to breathe. I saw an improvement that continued and anytime he gets sick, I take him there."**

Renee has an arsenal of strategies to keep her boys well. Combined with the salt therapy, she has salt lamps in their rooms and homeopathic drops on hand. She has started using aromatherapy oils and is also taking the boys to a kinesiologist* to help them deal with blocks from past trauma as well as the constant leg pain that Jake has from Sever's disease, a common cause of heel pain in childhood and early adolescence.

> **"Sometimes people think I'm weird and ask, 'What are you doing now?' I don't want my children to suffer or to be unhappy or to struggle. I think there's always an answer, but you have to go and look for it."**

I asked Renee what advice she would give to parents going through challenges with their children's physical or emotional health.

> **"Don't accept that it's just the way it is. There are things out there, there's help. Find that person that will support you or that medicine or that option. I don't think that one doctor can just dictate that. Don't accept that you're going to have to deal with that forever. Be open to alternatives that might seem weird or not the norm. Don't give up."**

When I caught up with Zac and Jake recently, it was hard to imagine Renee and Tim's challenges with them as babies. As the boys enter their teen years, their blessing is to have parents who prioritise their happiness and well-being.

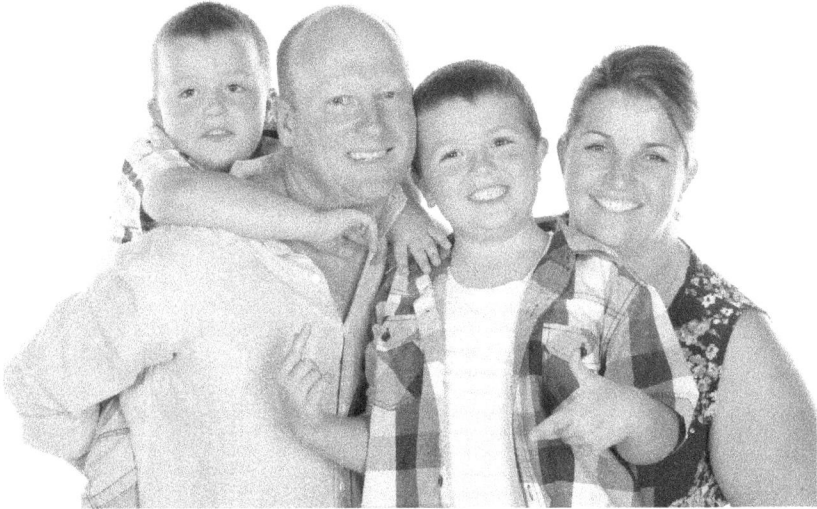

Jake, Tim, Zac and Renee

"Don't isolate yourself. Find your people. It might not be your family or your best friend. I've met lots of people through groups and some will get you through that time. You don't need to be friends with everyone you meet forever. Just keep meeting people and you'll either connect or you won't, trust that you'll know."

13

ADELE

- Three Miscarriages
- Postnatal Depression (PND)
- Postnatal Anxiety
- Rainbow baby, Eve, aged six
- Rainbow baby, Basil, aged one

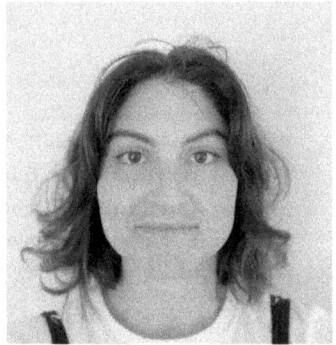

As the child of ex-patriot Brits living in Hong Kong, Adele had both western and eastern cultural influences in her early life. She returned to boarding school in England at the age of 14 and satisfied her scientific and creative talents by studying art, then medical microbiology.

It was an Australian who won Adele's heart. Following a 10-year career as a professional cyclist, Peter met Adele when they were both working in a London hospital.

> **"We got married in St Lucia in the Caribbean and wanted time together as a couple to kind of grow bored of each other, before we had children."**

Peter and Adele took advantage of their proximity to Europe and enjoyed travel to Spain, Italy and Egypt.

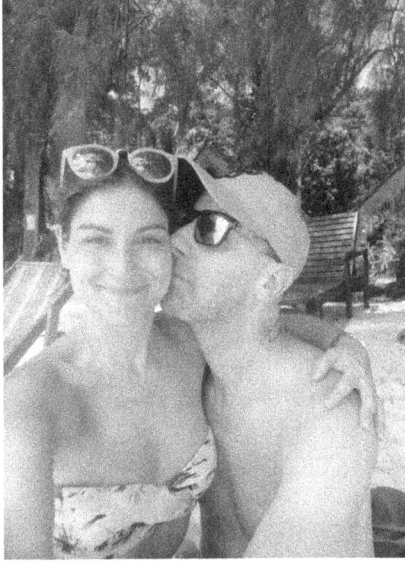

Adele and Peter

After a few years together, the couple began to think about starting a family and decided that Australia would be the best place to raise their children.

Adele's field of work was very specific—she was a scientist who developed new diagnostic tests for viruses and bacteria. It was important that they find a position that called for her particular skills. She was fortunate to secure a role with the right fit in Melbourne, paving the way for immigration in 2010.

After two years, Adele and Peter felt settled in their new city and decided that the time was right to have children. At the age of 29, Adele fell pregnant and everything was going to plan.

"My whole life, I've been fascinated with pregnancy and pregnant bellies. I've got two older half-sisters and four nieces and nephews. Every time there's a belly, I just want to touch it, talk to it and to feel the baby kick. And so, for me, being pregnant was really special and amazing. It was something I really looked forward to, and something I honoured because we really, really wanted it."

Five weeks into the pregnancy, Adele started spotting and cramping. She went to her GP and suspecting a miscarriage, he referred her to the Early Pregnancy Assessment Clinic.

Adele recalls her appointment at the Clinic as an awful experience. The couple arrived to find more than 60 people waiting to be seen before them. They took a number, sat down and then waited for hours.

> **"When we were called, this doctor just gets me on the table and says, 'Legs apart', and he starts going. My husband's like, 'Hang on a minute. What are you doing? You haven't even asked her permission.' We both work in healthcare and he worked in complaints and governance in the UK. The doctor said, 'We're taking swabs. Yeah, you've got a miscarriage.' And that's it. I'm just devastated. Nobody said sorry. Nobody said what caused it or how to recover. It was something so traumatic happening to me and I wasn't cared for properly. I felt really dirty afterwards."**

It was the worst possible scenario for Adele—she was given confirmation of her loss without any consideration for her emotional wellbeing. And on top of that, her physical body was subjected to an invasive procedure, without her permission, and with dubious relevance.

The couple left with neither information on what to expect, nor avenues for support. Well-meaning friends and family tried to be supportive, but some of their comments were dismissive of how the trauma affected Adele.

> **"I think what was most hurtful was a conversation with my mum about it and she said, 'Oh, it's very common.' That's what a lot of people would say. I don't care if it's common. It's still painful. We all die at some point, but at someone's funeral, you don't say, 'It's very common that we die. You shouldn't be feeling sad, it's common.' That completely disregards the emotion."**

Adele had already imagined her child and what her family would look like. She had already imagined everything she hoped for her baby's future and in an instant, it vanished. Having been able to direct and manage most of the other elements in her life, Adele found it frustrating that this was a process that she could not control.

> **"It felt like a kind of misfire, the devastation where you're on a path and suddenly, you realise you have to go back two steps and start again with a little hole in your heart for what could have been."**

Her psychologist was a great help during this time. Adele has suffered from depression and anxiety since she was 18. At different periods of her life she had been on medication, but prior to her miscarriage, Adele had been well for several years. The psychologist helped her to deal with her emotions, encouraging her to cry as much as she needed. Adele worked through her pain, reframing the loss by thinking about "a little soul up there, just waiting, waiting for me."

There was no definitive reason for why her miscarriage had occurred. Adele questioned her own fitness and health, wondering if there was something physically wrong with her. She examined their diet and lifestyle, and on that basis, it did not make sense. They ate healthy food and mostly cooked from scratch. They did not drink alcohol or take drugs. They were both active and of a healthy weight. There was nothing that appeared to be wrong, so after six months, they decided to try again.

Adele feels highly in tune with her body and has found that she instinctively knows when she is pregnant. She is almost 100% sure that her second pregnancy was conceived on a trip to England for a friend's wedding.

From their previous experience, the couple had little faith in the public health system, and this time they engaged a private obstetrician. At seven weeks pregnant, Adele had the faintest pink spot and called the doctor's emergency number. The couple went to have a scan and discovered that the ovum had not developed properly. Again, they were faced with disappointment, but it made a huge difference that the doctor was sympathetic and provided specific instructions on what would occur next. She gave Adele some medication to speed up the miscarriage, and explained that it would be better than having a D & C.

"It was quite a lot of cramping, very painful but pretty much over within a day. When it starts happening, you just want it to be over so you can try and regroup and try again."

Once Adele felt well enough, the couple made a decision that was completely out of character. Instead of moping about at home, they went out to a cocktail bar and took it in turns to order cocktails for each other.

"We were commiserating the loss of our baby. And we shared memories of our relationship and laughed. We got drunk. We were silly. We just had fun, the two of us. It was a beautiful way to get over it, or get through it, together."

Peter also felt the loss. Being 13 years older than Adele, he was just as keen to start their family, but at the same time, the miscarriages made him feel hesitant about another attempt because it would mean going through the pain all over again.

"They're so powerless, the men. It's a grieving process for them too. They've also lost a child, and on top of that, they're having to be strong for us while we're physically going through it."

Adele didn't want to go through the pain again either. Her scientific mind questioned the futility of just trying again without finding out what was wrong. She needed to uncover the problem and resolve it.

With the medical profession unable to provide any solution, Adele turned to Chinese medicine. The couple went to a traditional Chinese herbalist and he asked questions about their health, including specifics about the colour of Adele's period. Hers had always been a dark red and through the consultation, she discovered that she had never had a proper period. Adele's womb was not being fully cleansed with each period—it was holding on to old blood and that meant that her womb lining was not fresh.

Adele started on a course of herbs and acupuncture, and a month later, she had her first bright red, fresh blood period. One month later, she instinctively felt she was pregnant and went to see her GP. He performed a test to confirm, but that came back negative.

"I told him I was really sure I was pregnant, and he said, 'I'm afraid not, you could try again.' He probably thought I was a crazy woman who wanted a baby so badly that I was having a phantom pregnancy. So, a week later, I tested and there was a faint line. I took a picture and emailed him with the words, 'I'm not crazy. I am pregnant.'"

Apart from dreadful morning sickness, the pregnancy progressed through each scan and check beautifully. I asked Adele about her emotional wellbeing during her pregnancy.

"I was pretty positive. I was doing a lot of yoga, a lot of prenatal yoga and visualisations with that. We found out we were having a girl and I could see her. I could see her in this garden, with black curly hair and pale skin."

At 38 weeks, the obstetrician felt that the baby was a little small and she asked Adele to go in for a scan the next morning. Up until that point, Adele had attended most appointments and scans by herself, but for this one, she asked Peter to attend. He literally said, "Do I have to come with you?" And when she said yes, he packed his bike into his car, plus a pile of old boxes that he intended to take to the dump later that day.

They left early to miss the peak hour traffic and waited an hour for the scan. Once they had the test, the sonographer asked them to wait a few moments and then she returned, informing them that she had phoned the hospital and that they should go straight over to the labour ward.

Adele's placenta appeared to be tight and it had reduced the blood flow to just 10%. The baby was not yet in distress, but they wanted to speed things along.

> **"I turned to my husband and said, 'You better get rid of those boxes and bike. And you need to bring my suitcase'. So, I'm in labour ward and he's doing errands because we're totally ill prepared. We had no idea this could happen."**

Peter had expected to leave the scan appointment and cycle to work. Instead, he was rushing in the opposite direction, dumping boxes, feeding the cat, grabbing the suitcase and driving back so he wouldn't miss his baby's birth.

Meanwhile, Adele had a drip inserted and was administered with Syntocinon*.

> **"I hadn't eaten anything. They wouldn't let me eat in case I had to have an emergency caesarean. It was very, very intense. I was not prepared for it at all. I was shaking, and of course, the lovely midwife goes, 'You've got a long way to go yet, love.' Oh, that helps. I said, 'Okay, epidural please.' After that it was a lot better."**

Eight hours later, Eve was born, a tiny 2.3kg girl.

The new family stayed in hospital for five days, including one extra day due to Adele's history of depression and anxiety. During that time, different midwives would offer all types of advice and Adele found it all overwhelming.

> **"I really struggled with all the conflicting advice. I probably shouldn't have stayed in that extra day because I got into a spin where I had so much advice that I didn't know what I wanted to**

do and what was the best thing. So, I would do this, and then I would try something else, I never knew what was right. I felt like I couldn't do it. I felt like a failure."

Adele compared herself with other new mothers and they all seemed to be able to cope whereas she was struggling. By the second night, Eve was sleeping all day and awake all night. Adele wasn't sleeping night or day.

They went home after the fifth day, and life continued in the same pattern. Then, their water heater broke and they had no hot water in the middle of winter. This added another layer of stress to an already tough situation. Eve was catnapping during breastfeeding, so that became a slow and difficult process. It was further complicated by Adele's commitment to following the instructions she was given at the hospital. Due to Eve's small size, Adele was told to wake her newborn if she was asleep at feeding time and to never allow her to sleep past four hours. This became a cycle of feeding, changing and putting Eve down to sleep, then resting for two hours before having to do it all over again.

No matter what they tried, they could not get the temperature of the room higher than 18 degrees and Eve felt so cold. They swaddled her, used extra blankets, but nothing warmed her. Eventually, Peter held her in his arms all night while sitting in a chair under a blanket, watching her sleep.

"I was getting depressed, Peter was depressed. The cat was wandering around wondering what the hell happened. It was just a nightmare."

Adele felt a huge pressure from the midwives to breastfeed, but after a few days, she could not continue.

"It was just torture. I never wanted to breastfeed. I hate it so much. And then when you make the decision to bottle feed, nobody tells you how much to give, what to do or how to clean the bottles because everyone's just pushing breastfeeding."

The child health nurse came for a home visit and commended Adele on the wonderful job she was doing. She inspected the house and nursery and told her to keep it up. The nurse only seemed to be interested in the baby, rather than the whole situation and the way in which motherhood was affecting Adele—the new mum was lying on the couch exhausted, unable to eat, drink or sleep.

The family was booked in for newborn photography at a studio the following day. The photographer took one look at them and saw that the new parents were shattered. She took the baby off their hands and told them to rest while she handled the photo session.

On their way home, Adele texted a special friend who she refers to as her "Australian mum." The text read:

> **"I've made a massive mistake. I can't do this. I need to give Eve up for adoption, or I need to leave."**

Her friend heard the desperation in Adele's message, and as a midwife and nurse, she realised that Adele needed help. She went straight over and after some research, they found a psychiatric hospital with a maternal child ward. Adele voluntarily admitted herself.

The staff took over the care of Eve and Peter was sent home to gather some things. He phoned some friends, breaking down in tears as he shared their situation. Peter returned and stayed with his family at the hospital, six days a week.

To help Adele on the path to wellness, the first step was to get her into a routine. She was given medications to help her sleep at the right times, and also to modify her serotonin levels. During the day, Adele would participate in programs to help her build a relationship with Eve. They also taught her how to look after her newborn without sacrificing her own wellbeing.

Step-by-step, Adele moved forward. As her confidence grew, she would go home during the day, then return to the safety of support at night. She gradually took over the night shifts with Eve and reached the stage when she felt able to cope on her own. Nine weeks later, Adele and Eve went home.

> **"The biggest kicker that I've struggled with for the last five years, has been wanting my baby so much and then being so depressed and unwell that I wanted to give her up for adoption, and struggling with that guilt."**

Adele and Eve returned to the hospital on a weekly basis to meet with other outpatients. They would join in the playgroup and this would give the mothers an opportunity to discuss how they were feeling and the difficulties they were facing. The hospital had an excellent program that focused on cognitive behavioural therapy. Adele attended classes and learnt useful relaxation techniques, mindfulness activities, and coping strategies. She learnt to rationalise her emotions instead of letting them run rampant.

Yoga became a vital part of Adele's wellness regime. She found teachers who would allow her to bring Eve, and sometimes mother and daughter would attend up to four times a week. Adele worked really hard on herself to become strong of mind and body.

> **"I worked on all sorts of goals and on being focused on more than just the end point. I started to focus more on the journey and the progression. I started to re-evaluate the way I've lived my life."**

Adele found that in the past, she would do and do and do until she crashed. She now tries to do less and to balance the doing with resting.

> **"It still happens a little bit, but the depths of the spikes are not so big. Peter helps me too. He says, 'You're doing too much today.' So, I have those different techniques and I also brought in meditation."**

When Eve was one year old, Adele went back to work for six months, but it was too much. The bullying at work and the juggle of family with the responsibilities of the job caused her mental health to suffer badly. Adele left the position and made working on herself and her bond with Eve her greatest priority.

Eve was growing well but she had developed a horrendous nappy rash that would not go away. Suspecting a dairy intolerance, they switched her to a soy baby formula. When the rash continued, they consulted their paediatrician who tested for infectious causes. The results were negative, so they asked if it could be the soy formula. The doctor confirmed that there was evidence that dairy and soy intolerances were linked.

Unable to solve the cause, Adele tried to treat the symptoms with every type of nappy rash cream on the market, but none of them worked. As her mother was an aromatherapist, Adele was familiar with essential oils and she wondered if there could be a solution that she could make.

Adele studied aromatherapy and with her scientific background, she produced a range of organic baby care products that are both effective and enjoyable to use. With the brand name, Honestly* the range includes a baby care box subscription, baby lotion bar, nappy balm and more.

Peter and Adele wanted another child, but there were mental barriers to overcome.

> **"Even though it happened with Eve in just seven days, enough damage had been done. It's taken me years to build up that**

bond and even now, I struggle with feeling insufficient. Especially because she has such a strong bond to my husband because he became the primary caregiver. That feeds my feelings of failure and inadequacy. That was a barrier to having another child, because you can see all that damage happening again."

Once Eve was four, the couple felt they were ready, and Adele fell pregnant while on a holiday to Thailand. She initially felt positive, but within about six or seven weeks, she felt an awful sense of dread. Her GP sent her off for a scan. The sonographer reassured her, saying that it was too early to tell what was happening and that they should let nature take its course for a few weeks then come back for another scan.

Adele convinced herself that everything was fine and went back a couple of weeks later. There was no heartbeat, even though the baby had grown a little. They were referred to the Early Pregnancy Clinic and after hours of waiting, another scan confirmed that loss.

"I couldn't get over the fact that nothing had happened. I had no real cramping. It was a missed miscarriage, and I think that is where I felt the most betrayed because I trusted my body to be in connection with me. It basically lied to me because my breasts were still large. They were still sore. I was still nauseous. I had all the pregnancy symptoms except I had no baby."

Adele was given the option to have a D & C, or to have medication to pass the tissue from her uterus. The staff suggested that the medication was not always effective, and recommended surgery. Adele followed the advice given and returned the following day for the procedure.

Even though she works in hospitals, Adele has never been a patient for anything other than pregnancies and birth. This was the first time she had ever experienced pre-op and post-op procedures, anaesthetic and theatre.

"The most traumatic thing was waking up in recovery, not really conscious, but in such a state of grief. I just started sobbing. I cried and cried and cried. It was the most awful thing. I was so scared and so alone, and then so sad."

She begged for her husband, but no visitors are allowed in the recovery room. Eventually someone fetched Peter and she was discharged into his care.

Three days later, Adele felt very sick and her GP diagnosed her with an infection. He prescribed strong antibiotics which she took for two weeks. This whole experience made her lose faith in the hospital system, and Adele sought out a Chinese medicine practitioner who was renowned for fertility. He provided her with treatment and within two months, Adele was pregnant.

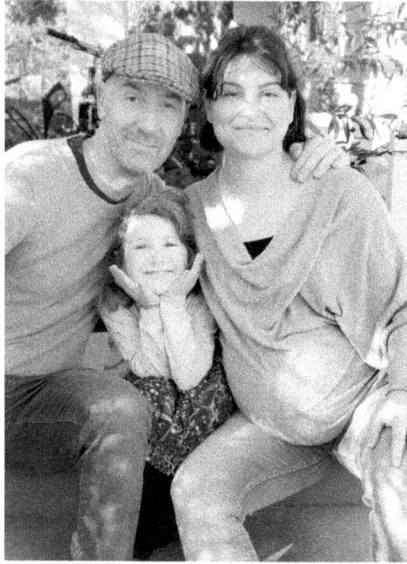

Peter, Eve and Adele

The couple sought a private obstetrician who was happy to be consulted anytime they had a concern. Adele attended fortnightly appointments, and all appeared well, with the baby kicking and active, though a little small. At 20 weeks, the baby was in the 70th percentile, by 30 weeks, down to the 50th percentile, and by 34 weeks, even further down to the 15th percentile.

Adele increased her visits to the hospital for twice weekly heart rate monitoring. At 38 weeks, the doctor recommended induction.

"He's like, 'Let's induce. We'll do the scrape*.' It's not a pleasant experience. I call it hardcore fingering."

Unfortunately, that did not work, so the doctor administered Syntocinon and an epidural. He tried the Foley bulb* to encourage dilation and then broke her waters. The baby was in the posterior* position causing awful pain in Adele's back, despite the epidural. The baby's heart rate dropped, and the delivery room was suddenly full of medical staff. Peter was shaking, and Adele was determined to get the baby out fast. Thankfully the baby turned, the doctor attached a ventouse vacuum and after six hours labour, Basil was born weighing 3.1kg.

Unlike their experience with Eve, Adele and Peter ensured that they were fully prepared for their second baby.

> **"I had been more in the sphere of pregnancy and infant loss. So that gave me quite a bit of fear, where before, I was really oblivious to that, I didn't know to be frightened. But this time I knew. Because of my history with postnatal depression, we were seeing a psychiatrist throughout my pregnancy. So we put everything into place. I had medication in my bag. As soon as the signs started to show, that was it, straight onto medication."**

Adele did try to breastfeed Basil. His latch was perfect, and he did well for a few days until Adele got sick. She did not want to fall into that same trap of feeling like a failure and transferred him to bottle feeding.

At the time of writing, Basil is one year old and thriving.

> **"I'm so happy with Basil, I'm enjoying him immensely. And I'm grateful that I can enjoy him."**

Eve is an adorable and happy six-year-old and the family is doing well. Adele continues to work on herself every day. She is aware of the signs of stress, and immediately implements the techniques and tools she has developed. And through her Honestly Store, Adele is using her personal experience and training to improve the lives of other mums and babies.

> **"Mothers are committing suicide. We've all seen that. There are some places they can go, but there are waiting lists. You cannot have waiting lists. You need help straight away—when it happens, it happens."**

14

REBECCA

- Declan, aged five
- Angel baby, Lucas
- Two Rainbow babies, Identical Twins, Chloe & Leah, aged one

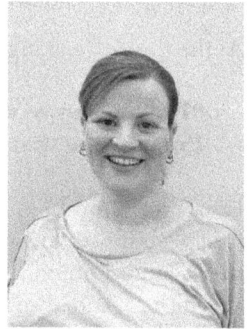

R ebecca and Toni met on ANZAC Day, one of Australia's most important national occasions. It marks the anniversary of the first major military action fought by the Australian and New Zealand Army Corps forces during the First World War.

They were both involved in a gambling game called two-up, played extensively by Australian soldiers and now enjoyed on ANZAC Day.

"She was spending all my money and I was trying to win it back," joked Toni. "Nothing has changed."

The couple dated for around eight months and all was going well until Toni noticed a lump in his neck. He went to the doctor who gave him a likely diagnosis of an infected or enlarged gland, but blood tests and a fine needle biopsy were arranged to be sure. The biopsy proved inconclusive because a sample could not be obtained, so Toni was advised to undergo surgery to have an incision biopsy*. The results came back, and Toni was diagnosed with lymphoma*.

"You don't expect these things when you're 25 years old,"
shared Toni. "Then I started getting the thoughts in my mind
that I'm going to die. That's the first thing you think of when
someone tells you you've got cancer. That's the first thing that
comes into your head.

So, from there, I had to take a few steps back and just start
looking at the bigger picture. What do I have to do to get
through this?"

Toni never considered that it would be something so serious. Throughout
the testing and right up until the surgeon gave him the diagnosis, Toni
thought he would be fine. But when the results came in, it hit him hard.

Cancer can be a huge stressor on a new relationship, but not for Rebecca
and Toni. Rebecca invited Toni to move in with her, so she could take care
of him throughout the four months of chemotherapy and two months of
radiation.

The treatment took its toll, with Toni experiencing the full effects of each
chemotherapy cycle, from the steroid high immediately after infusion,
followed by the low of no energy, then the gradual building up of white
blood cells before the next dose hit again.

Toni is grateful that his specialist fully informed him of the risks to fertility
that could be caused by the cancer treatment. He was told that between 10
and 20 per cent of men become infertile, and as he was a young man, the
specialist sent him to deposit at the sperm bank just in case he needed it in
the future.

Fortunately, Toni's cancer treatment was successful, and he has been well
ever since. After four years together, he proposed to Rebecca and they
married two years later.

The couple had always wanted children and Rebecca fell pregnant
naturally in early 2014. The pregnancy progressed well, though the birth
was dramatic.

"It was about 26 hours labour, a lot of hours. It was intense.
Especially for a first baby, you have no idea! I wasn't dilating,
and they put on the monitor and he was going into distress.
They said I had to have a caesar. I went into shock because
that's not what I planned to have, but when they said that's the
way it's got to be, I said, 'okay.'"

Rebecca was given an epidural shortly before baby went into distress. This
step provided the perfect preparation for surgery, enabling her to be taken

to theatre immediately for an emergency caesarean. Soon after, Declan was born, a healthy and happy boy.

The couple enjoyed raising Declan over the next couple of years before deciding to add to their family. Again, they conceived without needing to use Toni's banked sperm.

At the 19-week ultrasound the sonographer was having trouble getting a good picture of the baby's heart. She asked Rebecca to move around and to return 20 minutes later for another try. At this point, the couple was not worried—the same thing had happened with Declan. Rebecca jumped around to get the baby moving but the sonographer was still unable to get a proper image, so she asked them to return the next day.

Toni was not available the following day, so Rebecca's sister accompanied her to the scan. After another attempt, Rebecca was informed that things weren't quite right. The sonographer said she would send the images to her obstetrician and advised her to book an appointment as soon as possible.

> **"I didn't think it was going to be anything bad. I just thought they were going to do an extra test or something."**

The obstetrician received the scans and explained that the sonographer had not been able to get a proper picture of the baby's heart and that it appeared that some valves were missing. Additionally, there was too much fluid in some parts of the brain and the brain structure was abnormal. In order to correctly diagnose the problem, the obstetrician asked to perform an amniocentesis.

> **"I thought something was not right but not to that extent," said Toni. "It hits you once you're in there, because what happened is, he said, 'Oh yeah, we're going to do an amniocentesis to get some cells out to test for genetics.' Then they put me in the corner, so I couldn't even do anything."**

Toni felt pushed aside during the procedure, and Rebecca would have loved to have him beside her. Nevertheless, the sample was procured, and the cells were sent off to be cultured.

In the meantime, their specialist sent them to the Royal Hospital for Women for more detailed ultrasounds, a heart scan, and a few other tests. Once the results came through, the professor who was caring for them offered a little hope.

"We found out he was a boy. The professor explained, 'He could just be a slow learner. He could be this, he could be that.' So, we thought, we can deal with that. If he's just got a bit of autism, it doesn't matter, we still want this baby."

The news made them feel better and a little more confident. It was a couple of days later that everything changed—the obstetrician received the amniocentesis results and found that the baby was missing the top and bottom of chromosome 18 known as 18p and 18q.

"He kept saying pathogenic. It was pathogenic. And I thought, what does that mean? I now know it is something that causes disease. He had the paperwork and there was list of possible things that could be the problem.

Some people can function with missing chromosomes, but more so in the middle, or you may have extras and that's okay. But our baby was missing the top and the bottom. It created a rare ring. They said it was too rare, that everything was rare with this."

They discovered that he was basically missing the important parts of the chromosome that fed the development of the heart and brain. There was the possibility of retardation and several different diseases. No one could say exactly how the baby would develop, all that could be provided was a least-to-most range of possibilities.

Rebecca and Toni were then presented with the most difficult decision they have ever had to make—whether or not to continue the pregnancy.

"They don't make a decision for you. They try to present all of the routes," explained Toni. "Then once everything was laid out to us, he said, 'Now you guys have to make a decision. What do you want to do? Do you want to continue with the pregnancy or not? It's up to you guys.' But he kept on saying, 'This is very rare and severe.'"

When babies are more than 20 weeks' gestation, it requires the approval of two medical practitioners to terminate. The couple asked about this and were informed that because they had been to the Royal Women's Hospital, in their case, there would be no problem whichever way they wished to go. He also told them that if they were to go down the route of continuing the pregnancy, it would be very traumatic.

"It was hard to cope with it because it was all just thrown at us. We spoke to the genetic counsellors and they said that if I was to fall pregnant again, this possibly wouldn't happen. It was just one of those rare things. The egg didn't split exactly in half and all those kinds of things. And the midwife up there, she was really lovely. She said, 'You've already got a son who's normal. There's nothing wrong with him. The chances are you'll be fine.'"

With all the information provided, the couple discussed the options and made their decision to terminate. Their obstetrician had planned a holiday for the following week, so they went back to see him a couple of days later. Once they had decided, they just wanted it done.

The doctors were helpful in fast-tracking the paperwork. It usually takes two weeks for approval, but they kindly processed it quickly. Every day the baby was getting bigger and since they had decided not to continue, every day they waited was more excruciating than the day before.

Three days before the induction, Rebecca took a tablet to get labour started. It worked effectively and she began to have pains. On arrival at the hospital, the staff prepared the couple for what was to come.

They explained that the baby might look deformed and broached the subject of what the couple would like to do after birth. Rebecca was asked if she would like to hold the baby, making it clear that it was completely her choice. They also asked Toni if he would like to cut the cord. The answer to both questions was yes.

At around 6.45am the doctor gave Rebecca a further labour-inducing medication. They broke her waters and Lucas was born at 1.34pm. Tears filled both Rebecca and Toni's eyes as they described those moments to me.

"Maybe it's the shock and trauma or everything else. I don't know whether it's just me, but I feel like every time I have a labour, I need to go to the toilet. I ended up having him on the toilet actually. They prepped for that fall and put the little dish in there and I kind of knew that's probably where I was going to be. So, we caught him, everything was fine and Toni still cut the cord."

The staff asked if they would like to stay, giving them space and time to bond with Lucas overnight. A support worker provided them with an angel gown outfit, but apart from that, they weren't given any further information on what to do. Up to that point, they had followed their doctor's instructions, step-by-step. Now that their baby was delivered, they were left to figure out the next steps on their own.

"I asked the support worker, 'Do we have to have a funeral?' And she said, 'Yes.' You'd think that she'd give us literature about stuff like that, something to help but I got nothing. I wasn't even prepared to stay that night. I was like, I'm having this baby then I'm going to leave that's it, done.

We didn't think to pack him clothes. We didn't think that we would be allowed to stay. We didn't know. Looking back now, I wonder, why don't they just lay it all out?"

Sadly, a cuddle cot was not provided, nor was a Heartfelt professional photographer organised.

"They knew we were coming in, they knew that I was 22 weeks by this stage, so everything should have been laid out and prepared. But it didn't seem like it was. It's different when you've gone full-term and something just happened. But for our circumstances, you would think that everything should have been mapped out and ready to go."

The couple took a few photos on their own phone, but Rebecca explained that she felt, "A bit weird, standing there taking photos of him. And to look at him and compare Declan as a baby, they were definitely brothers." A midwife took some photos and they are grateful that she captured those special moments before they left the hospital.

"Walking out that corridor without Lucas was the hardest, because with Declan, we took him home. This time, we got nothing."

Even though Declan was just three years old, he had an awareness beyond his years. Toni and Rebecca knew he would be expecting a baby and had no idea how to tell him what had happened. During the pregnancy, once they knew Lucas' condition, they tried to prepare him by saying that the baby was sick.

"He would just look at my belly and say, 'Baby's sick,' and then pat my belly. It was hard because you just didn't know what was going through his head, and you don't want to tell him much because you don't want to upset him."

Declan stayed with Rebecca's parents during the delivery, and when they returned home to him, he went straight to her belly.

> **"He just knew the baby was gone. I thought, how does he know this? We didn't take him to hospital because we thought it would probably be a bit too much because he's such a sensitive kid, so best not to go down that line. So, when we came home, he just patted my stomach. I didn't have to say anything, he just knew."**

Every now and again, Declan still asks about Lucas and they say he is up with the stars in heaven.

Toni and Rebecca focussed their energies on Declan. Having him really helped them to be grateful for the family they did have, rather than dwelling on what could have been. They also found their local support group for baby and child loss. Connecting with other families who had also experienced loss was helpful for them to come to terms with their own loss.

Two years later, the couple felt ready to try again and they were thrilled when they discovered that Rebecca was pregnant with twins!

The pregnancy proceeded beautifully with ultrasounds showing that the babies measured well. Apart from heartburn, Rebecca felt lucky to have normal blood pressure. Day by day, her belly became heavier more quickly than before.

At 34 weeks, Rebecca's labour pains started at 2.30am. The doctor had her booked in for an elective c-section at the 38-week mark, so Rebecca thought she had plenty of time to pack a bag. Her babies had other ideas, and in those wee hours of the morning, she threw a few clothes in a bag and rushed to hospital.

They admitted her immediately and administered medication to stop the labour. They ran some tests and monitored the babies for changes. The medication worked, and Rebecca was allowed to return home, with strict instructions to take things easy until the twins were delivered.

At the end of that week, Rebecca went to her standing obstetrician's appointment. Due to the preterm labour*, the doctor brought forward the c-section date by two weeks. Rebecca did well to keep the babies until the theatre date and went in to deliver as scheduled.

On the 7th November, Chloe Louise and Leah Grace entered the world, two healthy girls weighing 2.49kg and 2.71kg respectively.

Rebecca and Toni feel so lucky and grateful that the girls did not require special care. They were able to enjoy those first few days in their hospital room together and then, to come home as a family.

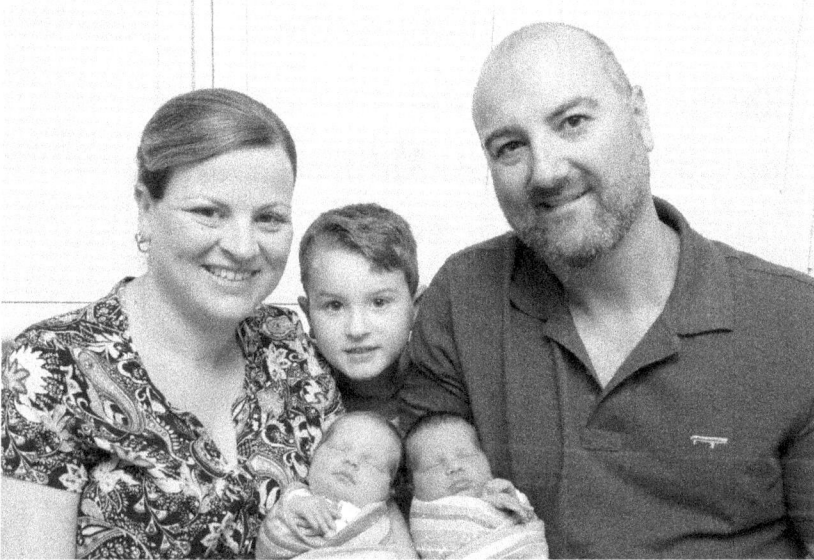

Rebecca, Declan, Toni and twins Chloe and Leah

15

JANE

- Multiple Missed Miscarriages
- Four Cycles of Unsuccessful IVF
- Intrauterine Insemination (IUI)
- Natural Killer Cells*
- Miscarriage
- Post-traumatic Stress Disorder (PTSD)
- Gestational Diabetes
- Carpel Tunnel Syndrome*
- Hannah, aged six months, Colic and Reflux

Special Note: Names and identifying details in this chapter have been changed to protect the privacy of individuals.

Jane grew up in the river city of Brisbane, a region of Australia known for its beautiful tropical temperatures and stunning coastline. After graduating from nursing, she decided to work abroad and traded her warm, sunny climate for the cold and rainy weather of London.

For around four years, Jane enjoyed the life of a young working single, fitting travel and social time around her nursing career. One night, some friends invited her out to see a band. It turned out that they knew one of the band members and that the band had invited quite a few of their friends to the event. One of those turned out to be her future husband, George.

"I flew out to India the next day and kind of forgot about him for a few weeks. Then when I got back, he rang me."

They dated for few months before Jane's visa ran out and she was forced to go home. George decided that distance was not going to keep them apart and, a few months later, he travelled to Brisbane for a holiday. He started discussing a more permanent move to Australia, but Jane was not ready for that.

"I freaked out a little bit and sent him back."

They continued separate lives with George returning to London and Jane deciding to study naturopathy. About five years later, the two reconnected by email and started talking about holidaying together and meeting up somewhere halfway. This didn't eventuate, with Jane deciding that this time, she would do the travelling. Her sister was now living in London and she flew over for visit. Inevitably, Jane and George did meet up again and six months later George left the UK to live with Jane in Australia.

Prior to George's arrival, Jane had started to think more seriously about starting her own family. At 34, she was well aware that biologically she was in the range where age becomes a significant factor.

"It's not that I was desperate to have babies at that stage, but I had it in the back of my head that there might be problems. I must have had intuition or something because I did go and see a gynaecologist just to check that everything was alright."

Her first experience with a gynaecologist was not just a waste of time, it was combative and disrespectful. Jane's request to be checked was dismissed with instructions to, "Start trying if you want to find out if you can have kids."

"I just wanted to know what my options were. Options like freezing eggs and that sort of thing which I probably would have done back then. It made me embarrassed to get another opinion because I thought, 'Maybe they all have that attitude.'"

When the doctor found out that Jane was a naturopath, the consultation deteriorated even further as the specialist proceeded to denigrate the therapy, arguing a case for why it was "rubbish". Needless to say, Jane did not bother to see this doctor again.

Three years later, George and Jane married and felt that they wanted to travel and enjoy their time together before having children. They did this for around 12 months and, when Jane turned 38, they were ready for a baby.

Jane did fall pregnant fairly quickly but then suffered a missed miscarriage after just a few weeks with a heavy, painful period. This happened two more times and, by then, she felt that there must be a problem and it was time to seek help.

> **"We weren't desperate to get pregnant, but just decided to try and see what happened. Then when we got pregnant straight away and started having miscarriage after miscarriage, we sort of started getting obsessed with it."**

After her last experience with a gynaecologist, Jane decided to go to a complementary* doctor to assist with fertility. Using a holistic approach, the practitioner diagnosed that factors such as age, stress, hormone imbalances and electromagnetic fields were affecting Jane's pregnancies. She tried various therapies, but the couple felt that they should also see a fertility specialist.

> **"The specialist didn't believe I was having miscarriages because I didn't have blood tests and scans as proof. So he tested George's sperm and did scans and tests on me. My Anti-Mullerian Hormone (AMH)* levels were really, really low."**

The AMH reading meant that Jane's viable eggs reserve was severely depleted. To encourage egg maturation during her cycle, the doctor prescribed hormone injections. He also implemented a technique called sperm washing* that was done before inserting the sperm in an IUI procedure.

The couple completed a few cycles using this method, but it did not yield the desired result. The medication had adversely affected Jane's hormone balance and the emotional toll was huge.

> **"I remember the day that the doctor said, 'You're never going to have kids.' I was absolutely devastated. How could he say that? He didn't how that for sure. I left his office and managed to get myself down to the car. I felt terrible, crying my eyes out."**

The doctor's opinion was delivered as fact. He had made a judgement that left Jane totally destroyed for months. She recalls thinking, "What's the point? Why do we keep trying? Why bother? It is what it is."

It was a tough time for Jane and George as they half-heartedly continued trying to conceive while dealing with their thoughts and emotions.

As time passed, they started to get angrier and angrier, changing their mindset and their view of that doctor's words from being fact to merely one person's opinion. They reminded themselves that it only takes one egg to make a baby and made the decision to find a new doctor.

Jane and George went to an IVF specialist and began the process of hormone injections again.

"I didn't respond well, and I didn't grow the eggs that I was supposed to, so they gave me more and more hormones. It was awful."

The scans showed that there was one egg growing and the goal was to nurture it until harvest. When the moment arrived, Jane went into theatre, fully expecting the egg to be retrieved, but when she woke in recovery, they told her that she had ovulated sooner than expected and therefore they were unable to procure the precious egg.

At this point, it was difficult to maintain a hopeful outlook, but a job offer to George in Sydney gave them the chance for a fresh start. They moved south and made an appointment with an IVF Clinic near their new home.

"It was just like a production line and they weren't really listening to what we were saying. It was the same thing—my body didn't respond. They were pushing it really hard and giving me more and more injections."

Jane was frustrated with the lack of interaction with the doctor. They were only dealing with nurses and she found that being denied direct and easy access to the specialist made it difficult to discuss her situation. When they reached the harvesting stage, Jane expected to get the call to come in for the procedure, but instead she received a call to say that her cycle was cancelled.

There was no explanation and it took a lot of chasing on the phone to finally speak to the doctor. He told Jane that he had looked at her hormone levels and it appeared that she was going to ovulate before they could harvest and that was why they decided not to go ahead.

"Why didn't he just tell me that? We were going to do another cycle with him and then decided that we didn't like the whole process, the way he was doing things."

With no results to show for all of the effort, physical toll and financial expense of seeing several fertility specialists, Jane decided to take a break and she was thrilled to find an amazing acupuncturist. She began with weekly appointments to assist with fertility, and at each visit the acupuncturist would assess Jane's needs, treating her nervous system, stress and any other issues to improve her wellbeing.

The acupuncturist also prepared a mixture of Chinese herbs as part of the treatment. After working with Jane for a few months, she suggested that natural killer cells could be the cause of her recurrent miscarriages and she provided the name of a doctor who specialised in this particular field.

Jane took up the offer and the couple made an appointment with the doctor who turned out to be another fertility specialist. The consultation became a repeat of their meeting with the first fertility doctor they had met.

"He asked, 'So were you actually pregnant? Do you know for sure? How did you know you were pregnant?' I said, 'I'm not here to argue whether or not I was pregnant. I'm wanting to investigate why I'm not getting pregnant.' I was about to run out the door crying.

And I saw George stiffening up next to me. I thought that I could either start crying or walk out the door. Or I could just give it to him. So I sat up and I said, 'Because I've done all my research and at this stage, I know what I'm talking about.' I gave him all the facts and all the research I'd done. He sat there and right then changed into a totally different person. He started talking to me with respect, like a human being."

From that moment on, the doctor treated them with consideration. Jane was happy with his change in behaviour but feels strongly that it is awful that women are frequently subjected to that type of attitude, especially at a consultation where they are already upset at their situation. She stressed that what women need from a doctor in those circumstances is compassion and understanding.

The specialist investigated Jane's level of natural killer cells and the results showed that she was a borderline case with insufficient problem cells to warrant treatment. He then devised a more tailored IVF program for the couple to try. They did two back-to-back IVF cycles with this doctor and, in hindsight, Jane feels that they probably should not have done them. Rather than responding positively, her body shut down completely.

They gave up on IVF after this experience and went on an overseas holiday to refresh and forget about tests and pregnancy for a while because it had consumed the last four years of their lives.

When they returned, Jane decided to only continue with her acupuncture treatments. The acupuncturist encouraged her to stay positive because she had helped other clients in similar situations to be become pregnant.

In 2018, Jane finally fell pregnant naturally. She was so excited, especially when she went for her blood test and first scan. The couple were absolutely thrilled to see their dreams coming true.

When Jane was seven weeks pregnant, George went overseas on a work trip. He was reluctant to leave, but Jane suggested that rather than staying home on her own, she would fly up to Brisbane and share the good news with her family personally. Jane was incredibly excited to tell her mum that she would be a grandma and the tears and celebrations were so joyful. But the excitement and expectation disappeared two days later when Jane miscarried in the middle of the night.

"It literally passed in the toilet, a sad, sorry little blob of an embryo. What was I supposed to do with it? That broke me. I pretty much lost hope. I became depressed and it affected my relationship with George because I was miserable, I was angry."

The loss was absolutely devastating for both Jane and George and they dealt with it in different ways. Jane had a post-traumatic stress response, with unexpected triggers causing her to break down in tears for seemingly no reason. She stayed in that dark place for several months, processing her trauma on her own, not wanting to talk to anyone about how she was feeling.

To make matters worse, they had just bought a home about an hour's drive south of Sydney, a place where they did not know anyone and were far away from friends and family.

"It was just me and my ball of misery, shutting George out. He was hurting as well. It was just as painful for him to talk about it. He's struggled because he's always said there's nothing for men in these sorts of circumstances. Women get limited support, but men just get kind of forgotten."

Eventually, Jane reached a place where she woke up one day and realised that she needed to get out of her rut. She joined a brunch group to meet new people and this helped her to slowly start socialising again.

These small steps gave Jane the lift to feel more like herself again. Even though they felt that the dream of one day having a child was slipping away, the couple still went through the motions of trying to conceive but without conscious expectation. They made plans as if they were never going to have a baby, instead pouring their time and energy into renovating their house.

Just a few days before Christmas day in 2018, Jane thought she had better do a test just in case she was pregnant because she was going to a few parties and did not want to be drinking if she happened to be pregnant. Jane could not believe it when it came back positive.

> **"I just had it in my head that it wasn't going to happen anymore. My whole thinking had to shift. I was so happy but so scared."**

Five weeks into the pregnancy, tests by Jane's GP showed that she had gestational diabetes. She was given a strict diet to follow for the remainder of the pregnancy.

At eight weeks' gestation, it was time for their first ultrasound. The couple were so relieved that everything looked great, but the feeling was short-lived when a few days later, Jane started spotting. She immediately became devastated, thinking that she had lost the baby again because that was approximately the same time her previous pregnancy had ended. But this time, the baby stayed.

> **"I was so highly anxious the whole time. Every time I went to the toilet I thought, 'Am I going to be bleeding?' I started a new job and wondered if working was going to kill it."**

The couple sought care from a different obstetrician near their new home, and he told them that their baby had a high-risk of Down Syndrome. Jane's age was associated with a one in eight chance. The doctor started talking the couple through their options, including additional tests and termination. He recommended that they consult a genetic counsellor for another opinion.

This information increased the couple's already heightened levels of anxiety. The genetic specialist outlined the dangers of the available tests, informing them about the risk of miscarriage with an amniocentesis* and the efficacy of the new Harmony test. They decided to go with the amniocentesis because they wanted to know for sure if the baby had the chromosomal indications of Down Syndrome.

"At the last minute, I was freaked out about the amniocentesis. I cancelled and said that I could not take that risk. It was too invasive. My intuition told me she was fine. We ended up doing the Harmony test and we had to wait 10 days for the result. When they phoned, I felt my heart skip a beat—I'd had too many of these phone calls."

It was good news—there was no need to fear the call because their baby was healthy, there were no sign of abnormalities and the expectant parents found out they were having a girl!

Jane's pregnancy reached 22 weeks, and she recounted how terrified she was during this period. Knowing that they needed to reach 24 weeks to be compatible with life, she felt desperate to meet that marker.

"I didn't have that wow, I'm pregnant feeling. I feel like I missed out a bit because I never had that joyful pregnancy without expecting something to go wrong."

At 24 weeks, the baby was doing well but Jane was suffering from high blood pressure. Her gestational diabetes had reached the stage where she needed to have regular insulin injections and she also started to swell. At 29 weeks Jane had to stop work and was advised to elevate her feet as often as possible.

The most troublesome issue was temporary carpal tunnel syndrome in both of her hands. It caused Jane to have limited hand movement making it difficult for her to do even the most basic tasks.

Ten days before her due date, Jane went into hospital for an elective caesarean. The doctor had hoped the pregnancy would make it to 34 weeks, so the extra four weeks were a bonus!

"The spinal anaesthetic was the one thing I was most terrified of. I was scared of getting paralysed because of all the stories I'd heard of what can happen. I was terrified of jumping during the injection because she kicked around a lot and I hoped she'd just stay still."

Despite her concern, the caesarean went smoothly with Hannah born a healthy baby. The only issue was the need to monitor the newborn's blood sugar levels due to the presence of gestational diabetes.

"It was a bit weird, because all of a sudden I heard the doctor say the words, 'Time of birth.' As a nurse, I freaked out

because I'm so used to hearing the words, 'Time of death.' I didn't know they said it at birth until I heard it then. I wasn't quite expecting that."

Hannah spent the first night in the Special Care Nursery for observation. The following day she had recovered well and was transferred to the ward to stay with her mother. As with any new mum, getting used to her new role was challenging but Jane had the added issue of not being able to use her hands because of the carpal tunnel syndrome, something that is still healing some six months later.

"We needed a lot of help because I had a caesarean and I couldn't use my hands. She wouldn't sleep at all and we were having a few problems with breastfeeding. The lactation consultant had broken her leg, so she wasn't available, and the nurses said they were too busy. They were not very helpful at all."

A series of mistakes and the lack of care made an already difficult situation even more frustrating. One time, a phlebotomist* came to take blood for a test and when Jane asked what it was for, it turned out that they had come to the wrong patient. Then another time, a nurse was to bring in some of Jane's expressed milk to top up Hannah's feed. She arrived, not with Jane's breast milk but a bottle full of someone else's milk. These incidences failed to instil confidence in the couple and on the fifth day, they decided to check themselves out early.

Once they were home, mother and baby mastered breastfeeding and Hannah is doing well at six months of age. She did, however, suffer quite badly from colic and reflux and if laid on her back, she would cough and wake herself up.

"We were worried that she was going to choke, and she just wouldn't sleep, so we slept in the lounge room for the first few weeks. We took turns holding her upright, sitting in a chair so she could sleep, but we didn't sleep."

George took three weeks off to help out which was wonderful but, when he went back to work, it became debilitating for Jane because she felt like she could not put her newborn down to sleep.

Eventually, something had to be done and when Hannah was five months old Jane took her to an Early Parenting Centre for five nights. The program helped immensely, and the family continues to work on developing a healthy routine.

Jane would like to have another baby.

"I spoke about it to George and he doesn't want to go through the whole thing again. He said that he just can't go through it again. He said he only just held on with this pregnancy."

It's a sensible choice because they know only too well that because Jane is now 43 years old, it puts them in a category that is extremely high-risk.

The family is a happy one and Hannah is George and Jane's miracle, the centre of their world. They enjoy every single moment with their gorgeous girl and, sooner or later, they will definitely get started on those home renovations!

"Don't be afraid to talk to people about it—you'd be surprised at how many people have been through or are currently going through the same experience. Just don't give up hope and trust your own intuition as well. Don't rely on what other people and every specialist tells you. Don't get too swayed by what you're being told. Go with your own gut instinct. But mainly, just don't lose hope. You just never know."

16

SALLY

- Ectopic pregnancy*
- Ruptured fallopian tube
- Internal haemorrhage
- Miscarriage
- Human Papillomavirus 16 and 18*

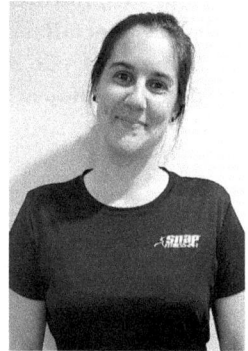

Flicking through the pages of tertiary education options after graduating from high school, Sally admits that she had no idea what she really wanted to do. Knowing that she loved the outdoors and adventure, her sister suggested a career in fitness and now 14 years later, Sally is an established body-positive fitness professional and speaker, helping people all over the world to achieve improved health and a better body image.

> **"Fitness sounded like something I didn't really have to think too much about. By the third day, I realised it was really cool and I loved it. I definitely didn't plan it but today I own my own business and have plans to open up my own studio. Things worked out really well."**

Sally's career gave her the flexibility to work to her own schedule in her home city of Brisbane. It also gave her the freedom to travel internationally to places as diverse as South America, Canada and several European countries including the Czech Republic and Austria.

"I was able to work as a fitness professional everywhere. That's given me a really interesting look at how we view health, fitness and body image in different cultures around the world."

While she was living Prague, an Australian client staying in their Austrian home invited Sally to come down for the weekend to enjoy a huge ski festival that was taking place in their tiny village. It was only a four-hour train journey away, so Sally decided to join them.

As they were walking through the crowd, her friend was carrying his skis and turned to talk to her. His skis hit a stranger in the head. His name was Dominik. It turns out that he was not only struck physically, but also soon became love-struck with Sally!

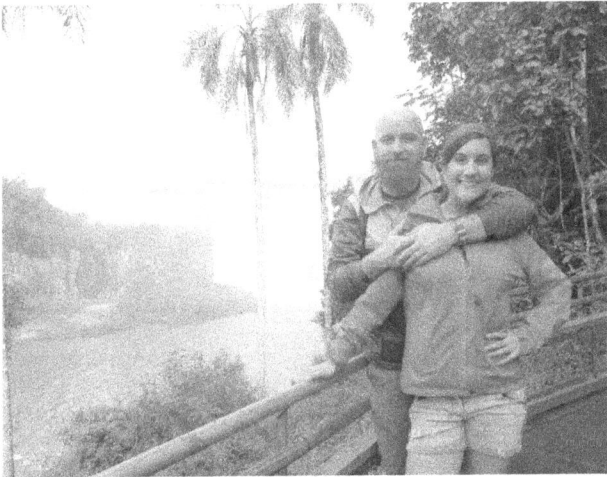

Dominik and Sally

The two started dating and within 18 months, the Australian and the Austrian were married. With travel and adventure on their minds, they took a 12-month honeymoon to South America before returning to Austria to live for a few more years.

Around the time that Sally was 30, the couple felt ready to start a family. They considered the best place to do that and made the decision to move to Australia.

"We always knew that we wanted to buy a house and have kids. It was really important to me that we did that here because I'm really close to my family. I have two sisters and my parents and we're all really close."

Dominik and Sally bought a house in a central location, around 20 minutes from centre of Brisbane and 20 minutes from Sally's parents. It needed to be renovated so the couple lived with Sally's parents while they worked on the house.

Having been on the pill for as long as she could remember, Sally was aware that it could take some time to fall pregnant, so they started trying to conceive. After just three months, she discovered she was expecting. She did the test around lunchtime and couldn't wait to tell Dominik.

"We were both really happy, but at the same time I said to him, 'Something's not right so don't get too excited.' It was a combination of pain, physical pain and just something in the back of my mind. That sixth sense."

As the day progressed, the pain continued to increase.

"I thought, 'I've never been pregnant before. Maybe this is a normal kind of pain.'"

With six clients scheduled for that evening, Sally did not want to let them down, so she headed into the gym. She lay down in the staff room for a minute and soon realised that something definitely wasn't right. There was no alternative but to cancel the clients and to drive home.

By the time she got into the car, she was experiencing waves of pain and each time one hit, she either braked or accelerated too hard. Thankfully, she reached home safely and went to bed. She noticed that if she lay very still, the pain would lessen.

"I think back and wonder why I was so hesitant to listen to what my body was telling me. Why? I think as women, we are very good at putting up with pain."

The following day, Sally rang her doctor who was happy to see her immediately. The GP performed an internal examination and said to Sally, "I don't want to alarm you, but I think you're having an ectopic pregnancy."

Sally had no idea what an ectopic pregnancy was, but she could tell by the doctor's response that it was something serious. The GP called the hospital emergency department and told them to expect her patient shortly. Sally was told to go directly to the hospital and to call her husband and ask him to meet her there.

When she arrived at the hospital, Sally was having trouble standing. As soon as the medical staff saw her, they brought out a wheelchair, sat her down and wheeled her past the 20 people in the waiting room.

A doctor came to her immediately with an ultrasound machine and commented that she appeared to have a lot of fluid. Sally was then promptly wheeled into another room.

"And then the next room I went into, eight medical people were in there and I thought, 'This is not normal.'"

By this time, Dominik had arrived and his support was exactly what she needed. One of the eight people explained that they had to do an internal ultrasound. The procedure was painful and invasive and once it was done, the medical staff conferred with each other and Sally was wheeled into another room. The couple were left alone with no information and only the staff's behaviour to surmise that there was something dreadfully wrong.

A short time later, one of the doctors came into the room and confirmed that Sally did have an ectopic pregnancy. Then he started saying that she would need surgery and kept talking about what had to happen, using medical jargon that made it difficult to understand.

"I was listening and thinking, 'What is happening?' And Dominik's first language is German. He speaks fluent English, but I had to just reiterate what the doctor was saying because he was stressed out. Obviously, he didn't know what was happening, he just knew it was bad. And when it's your second language, it's a lot harder to take things in, no matter how fluent you are."

It was a traumatic situation where Sally was trying to process the impact of the diagnosis and treatment herself, while trying to ensure that her husband also understood what was being said. More than anything, the thing she really wanted to know was if her baby was going to survive.

"I didn't know how to say it. But I said, 'Will it survive?' I didn't know if I should call it a baby. It was all so fast and such a shock. I thought that maybe if I don't refer to it as a baby, it won't be so hard. And he said, 'Oh, it's incompatible with life.' And I said, 'So that's a no?' And he said, 'Yes.'"

Sally was frustrated with the complex language being used throughout the entire discussion. Yes, she knew what the phrase, 'incompatible with life' meant and so did Dominik, but it felt like the doctor was making the situation even more difficult than it needed to be by not speaking plainly.

"Why do they make it sound so complicated? Why don't they say, 'No, he is going to die,' or, 'Yes, he'll be fine.'"

The scans had revealed that the fertilised egg was not in Sally's uterus, it was located in her right fallopian tube. This part of a woman's body is usually less than one centimetre in diameter so as the egg grew, it stretched the fallopian tube. This was the cause of her immense pain. Eventually there was so much pressure that the egg ruptured her fallopian tube causing internal bleeding. The doctors estimated that Sally had been bleeding for around 18 hours, haemorrhaging over 700 millilitres of blood.

Death can be caused by internal bleeding, and Sally's condition could have been fatal if she had not gone to hospital.

"I asked the doctor what would have happened if I had just kept on soldiering on for the rest of the day. He said, 'Well the situation would be very different.' I asked, 'Would I have died?' He said, 'Possibly.'"

The experience has taught Sally to listen to her body, and this is something she advocates strongly to her clients. She has found that the majority of women that she works with have a higher pain threshold than men, that women become used to pain as part of their life as they cope with monthly period pain, childbirth and more.

Sally has a much greater appreciation for the way her body communicates and encourages women to stop downplaying pain and to give themselves permission to go and seek help.

Even though she now realises that she probably should have gone to the doctor the previous day, Sally's decision to reach out for medical help immediately that morning in all likelihood, saved her life.

The doctor informed Sally that she would need salpingectomy* surgery immediately because every moment they waited placed her in more danger. She barely had time to ask Dominik to call her father before she was whisked away to be prepped for theatre.

Just before they went in, a doctor asked Sally if she would allow student doctors to observe. Thinking of the greater good, Sally agreed, but when they arrived she felt uncomfortable and changed her mind, but because she had already given her consent she did not feel that she could ask them to leave. Fortunately, a kind and nurturing nurse ensured she had a couple of minutes alone before the anaesthetic was administered and this calmed her down.

The procedure was done by keyhole surgery and involved excising Sally's right fallopian tube and cleaning out the pooled blood from around her organs. She still retains both of her ovaries and the only external scars are two small incisions on her left side.

Dominik was told that the surgery would take about half an hour, but it ended up lasting two hours.

> **"He said it was the worst two hours of his life. Half an hour would have gone by and his mind must have been wondering what was going on. It was a lot longer than it should have been because it was such a mess in there."**

The operation was successful, but recovery was slow. The gas they had used to expand Sally's stomach took a few days to dissipate and she felt physically uncomfortable. There was pain and difficulty with lifting and twisting movements, but the most difficult part was the way she felt.

> **"Emotionally, I was really disconnected. A grief counsellor came in the next day. She asked me a few questions and that was it. I went to my GP about a week or two later and she offered to send me to grief counselling but I said, 'I've been pretty sad. I'm still physically recovering but I think I'm okay.'"**

For the first few weeks after surgery, Sally was emotionally numb while dealing with the physical side of recovery. About a month later, something changed. On reflection, she is not sure what triggered it, but she remembers thinking, "I'm not okay."

Dominik and Sally took up an offer from Sally's aunt and uncle to stay in their holiday home on the south coast for a few days. It gave them a chance to take some time out and process what had happened.

> **"A good friend of mine who had a miscarriage the year before me suggested I write a letter. I decided that he was a boy. Obviously, we didn't know but it just felt right. I decided to name him Thomas. I found that helpful."**

Sally wrote the letter and the couple went together to the beach at sunrise. She read the letter out loud and then together they placed some flowers in the water and let them go. It was a way to honour their baby and a beautiful memory they will always share.

Sally's emotional state ebbed and flowed and around six months later, she started to question herself.

> **"One minute I was fine, everything was normal. Then I would think, 'How am I going to get through this?'"**

The support of family and her close group of friends played a major part in helping Sally during this tough time. Even though most of them had not experienced miscarriage, the fact that they were there for her was priceless. Sally also found support in miscarriage Facebook groups that connected her to other women who had been through similar experiences.

> **"I found that to be really helpful, knowing that you're not alone in feeling what you're feeling and knowing that it's okay to feel anything that you're feeling."**

Dominik also had his ups and downs, but not as intensely as Sally. He has always wanted to have children and began talking about it just three months after the couple met. Sally recalls how excited he was when she told him she was pregnant and then not 24 hours later, the excitement turned to intense fear about whether or not his wife was going to live or die.

Some months later when he returned to Austria for work, Dominik talked to his mother and also two friends whose wives had experienced miscarriages. Sally later learnt that Dominik had not talked to her earlier on because he thought she had "enough on her plate."

> **"He's been really supportive. He also views it as his son died. We've had conversations about that. He's told me that it's made him think a little bit about his faith. He's mostly been fine, but I don't know. It definitely affected him more than I thought."**

After around 10 months, Sally still didn't feel right and realised that she needed professional help, so she began seeing a psychologist.

> **"I thought I shouldn't be feeling this sad because other women have it so much worse. I was hung up on the whole idea that I can't be this sad because I lost him very early. I just couldn't stop comparing my grief which seemed like it should be less than other women."**

Sally also held guilt about her life—she was healthy, she had a family that loved her, she had the benefit of a private school education, she had worked hard and felt that she had a privileged life. This was the only bad thing that had ever happened to her so in a strange way, she didn't feel like she had the right to feel sad.

The psychologist helped Sally to change her thinking, showing her that she did not need to see things that way. She provided Sally with some practical tools such as writing her thoughts down, talking to Dominik about her feeling and to being kind with herself.

> **"She gave me permission and that's what I needed. I needed someone else to tell me that it was okay for me to just lie in bed sometimes. Because as a fitness professional, I'm always the one giving positive, uplifting energy to others."**

Apart from being a body fitness professional, Sally is also a trek leader and adventure trainer. She leads groups on what is regarded as one of the most physically and mentally demanding treks in the world—the Kokoda Track in Papua New Guinea.

As an expert in helping others to overcome challenges, Sally's expectations of herself were high and she admits that the past 12 months have been hard, but that there have also been rewards.

> **"It's allowed me to become more compassionate because you truly don't know other people's stories. It's allowed me to become more compassionate to myself. It's definitely the hardest thing emotionally to find a space and be kind to myself without letting my business fall down the drain."**

Another unexpected benefit was a deeper relationship with her clients. Most of the people Sally works with are women, and as she shared her story with them, the support was incredibly nurturing. It bonded the women together and gave Sally the sense that they were looking after her as much as she was helping them.

> **"When I shared with my clients, a good half of them said, 'Yes, I understand. I had a miscarriage.' There is a certain strength that I think you can derive in knowing that we're all in it together. As sombre as that is, it's going to happen, whether or not we share our experiences."**

In early 2020, Sally was diagnosed with HPV 16 and 18, the cause of 70% of cervical cancers and pre-cancerous lesions. She has undergone a successful LLETZ surgery to remove the abnormal cells and the couple is now ready to start trying to conceive.

> **"I'm feeling 80% positive and 20%, a little worried. What if it happens again? What if I just have a standard miscarriage? Generally, I'm the kind of person that feels the fear and does it anyway. It's not going to put me off trying again. We just hope it happens."**

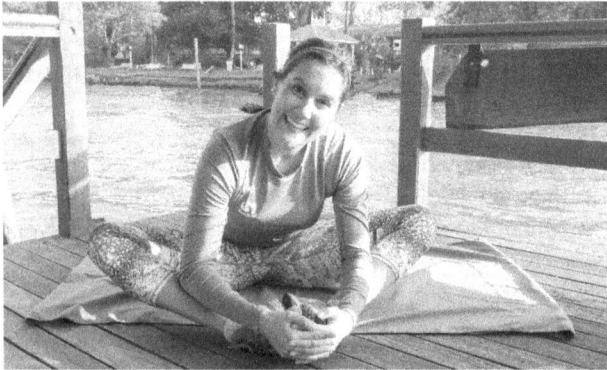

> **"I think that I have a certain responsibility as a person who's in a leadership position, to facilitate the healing of others. Because that's part of my job, and that's what I'm good at. And that's what I want to do. I have taken this experience as something that I hope I can help other women deal with."**

17

JESS

- Endometriosis
- Polymyalgia*
- Irritable Bladder
- Menstrual Migraines
- Hormone Treatment
- Cyst and Laparoscopy during pregnancy
- Pelvic Instability
- Harvey, aged six, Asyncliticism*, Tongue-tie*, Grommets*, Obstructive Sleep Apnoea*
- Post Birth Haemorrhage
- Endometriomas*
- Miscarriage
- Medically Managed Miscarriage*
- Subchorionic Hematoma*
- Violet, aged two

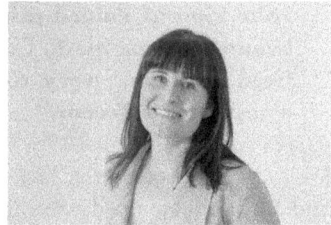

Jess grew up in the Adelaide Hills, a region known for producing excellent wines. It is also the site of Australia's oldest surviving German settlement, dating back to the 1830s. Located just 30km from South Australia's capital city, Adelaide, the area has retained a strong sense of community.

"All my family is still there—they all live on the same street. It's like a small country town."

Upon graduating from high school, Jess enrolled in a course to become a massage therapist. She thoroughly enjoyed learning and practicing the techniques but found some clients to be challenging.

> **"I really struggled when I had my own clients because I just couldn't go to the depth that men needed. Then when I had a female client, they'd say, 'How can I take you home? Oh, that was wonderful.' I was only 18 and I interpreted that as, I can't do this because I can't just say that I don't want to work with men, that's discrimination."**

With this in mind, Jess researched careers to figure out what she could do. She settled on midwifery and began her degree which involved learning the theory as well as the practical aspects of childbirth. Her first assignment was to interview a midwife. The woman she was referred to turned out to be a specialist in home births and Jess was invited to attend one of the midwife's deliveries.

> **"She kind of ruined midwifery for me because I went to this beautiful home birth. I thought, 'Oh, this is what birth is.' And from then on, every time I worked in the hospital, it was completely different."**

Jess was so upset by the lack of informed consent during hospital labour and birth that halfway through her degree, she changed to vet nursing. This was a profession she loved, being a bit of a self-confessed crazy dog person! Jess worked at a vet clinic for around eight years and it was during this time that she married her high school sweetheart, Simon.

Originally interested in her best friend, Simon asked Jess to help him arrange a date. It turned out that the two were not compatible, but it paved the way for Simon and Jess to become friends. They dated throughout university and married in 2011.

The newlyweds had arranged a honeymoon to Cuba with plans to start a family upon their return. Jess was advised that once she stopped taking her contraceptive pill, her normal cycle would return, and she would likely fall pregnant within a few months. But after a year, they were no closer to conceiving.

Clues to her inability to conceive can perhaps be discovered by looking at the symptoms Jess developed in childhood. She started her periods at the age of nine and the early onset of puberty caused her to develop acne. Her periods were extremely painful, something that her mother had never experienced. The doctor prescribed the contraceptive pill as a solution and it did lessen the severity of the pain. By the time she stopped taking it, Jess had been on the pill for more than half her life.

The contraceptive had appeared to balance her hormone issues, but in her 20s, Jess started experiencing episodes of extreme body pain.

"It would migrate around my body. One day my neck would be so sore I couldn't turn it, and the next day it would be completely better, but the pain would have travelled to a different part of my body. I was so lethargic. It was probably glandular fever."

Blood tests came back as negative for fibromyalgia*, an autoimmune disease*, though her inflammation levels were around eight times higher than normal. The medical diagnosis was polymyalgia*. Her doctor prescribed anti-inflammatory medication, but her sensitive gut reacted badly, and it made her nauseous. The only thing she could tolerate was Paracetamol and that did little to stop the pain.

With no effective treatment offered by medical doctors, Jess sought the help of a naturopath. Using a Vega* machine for diagnosis, the therapist looked at the results and asked, "Does anyone in your family have endometriosis?"

"No one in my family had any problems having children. My mum got pregnant with me even though she had a copper IUD and I'm the youngest of four children. When the naturopath said that I was like, 'Oh my god, that causes infertility.'"

Jess told her that she didn't think there was endometriosis in the family, so they moved on to the issues of lethargy and pain.

Two years later when Jess was trying to conceive, the memory of that consultation resurfaced when month after month, her period confirmed that she was not pregnant. The other issue was the pain—now that she was off the pill, the intense cramping was no longer masked by the medication and it became increasingly worse with every cycle. It got to the point when she was in pain almost every day.

Another issue arose that complicated Jess's health further—she developed chronic diarrhoea and was sent to a gastroenterologist*. He performed an endoscopy* and a colonoscopy* and these examinations did not yield insight into the cause. The specialist suggested that she might have Irritable Bowel Syndrome (IBS)*.

Unsatisfied with the diagnosis, Jess knew she had to keep searching for answers. The naturopath's question about endometriosis still played on her mind, so she asked her GP for a referral to a gynaecologist. There was a four month wait for an appointment, so in the interim she reached out to a gynaecologist she had met when she was studying midwifery.

"I went and saw this guy. I knew I wasn't going to get a lovely gentle bedside manner, but I was so desperate. He said, 'I don't think you've got it.' One of the symptoms I was having was pain during sex, which is not conducive to making a baby. And his response was, 'Well how long have you two been sleeping together?'"

Jess couldn't believe the gynaecologist's attitude. He failed to provide any answers and had belittled her in the process. Hoping for a better diagnosis, Jess went to her scheduled appointment at the gynaecologist she had been referred to by her GP.

"The only thing she asked me was, 'Where are you in your cycle?' I told her that I was around ovulation. She told me that even if my period was due tomorrow, that it was so thick and disgusting in there [uterus] that no one [embryo]would want to live in there."

The gynaecologist recommended a laparoscopy to offer a definitive diagnosis. She told Jess that if she had endometriosis, then she would need to stay the night in hospital. If not, she would be able to go home that night.

Following that surgery, Jess was informed that she would need an overnight stay and she had to wait until the doctor came in the following morning to receive her diagnosis.

"She said there was quite a lot of endometriosis in there. At my post-op appointment a month later, she casually informed me that they did a D & C while they were there and put dye through my tubes to make sure they weren't blocked. They were fine. Apparently, the D & C was supposed to help with implantation but none of that was explained to me."

The gynaecologist added that this would be the couple's best opportunity to conceive naturally. "You've got three months," she stated factually. "If you can't in that time, then you need IVF. But don't worry, I can help you with that."

Jess had a visceral reaction to her comment about requiring IVF after three months because it seemed that her motivation for the short timeframe was to move them swiftly into a program where she would make thousands of dollars in profit. The couple immediately sought a second opinion and booked an appointment with the leading endometriosis doctor in Adelaide. As expected, there were no appointments available for five months. It was a difficult wait for Jess as she was still experiencing pain despite the surgery.

"When you've had pain for a long time and it is not managed properly, your nerves start to get confused about what's painful and what isn't painful. It got to the point where I couldn't even sit down on a chair or anywhere without being in excruciating pain because my nerves were just so ready to fire off about anything."

Jess researched everything she could about endometriosis, pain management and fertility. One of the things she found was a book about menstrual cycle sequencing yoga.

"You do certain poses at different times of your cycle. I was getting so much pain relief by practicing yoga for one hour every night. That's where the rabbit hole of alternative health started."

In addition to the naturopath she was seeing regularly, Jess tried other therapies to help her manage her day-to-day pain and to increase her fertility. She started regular acupuncture by a practitioner who was also a Chinese herbalist, as well as chiropractic care.

After a five-month wait, the couple finally went to their appointment with the gynaecologist who they hoped would offer a solution. They walked into her office and saw that she had Jess's file from the other gynaecologist.

The doctor went through the file notes and commented that the previous specialist had written that Jess's uterine lining was thick and that rather than completely coming away and leaving a fresh lining for an embryo to implant, her lining was continually building up month after month. The doctor explained that Jess might have conceived many times, but the embryo had never implanted.

Jess could not believe that the other gynaecologist had written these notes but failed to disclose any of these facts to her. It further supported their conclusion that the previous gynaecologist had wanted them to become her IVF clients.

The doctor they were now sitting with was of the opinion that three months had been too short a timeline.

"She said, I think you should try for six months and then after that we might look at some fertility treatment. Let's try and shed that lining and get to a place where a baby will want to implant."

Jess explained that she had just started a new herb prescribed by her naturopath called Vitex, a product that helps your body produce more progesterone. Unexpectedly, the doctor said, "Oh, I quite like Vitex." The fact that the doctor knew about the supplement and was in favour of it gave the couple confidence that they were being cared for by the right person—a medical expert at the top of her field who was open to a holistic view of treatment.

They left that appointment with eight prescriptions and a plan for the next six months.

"I had a nasal spray for menstrual migraines and an anti-inflammatory that made me nauseous. Then I had an antacid to help with the nausea. Then I had a suppository anti-inflammatory and I had just one and it gave me diarrhoea. My body was like, 'Get it out!' Then I had Mersyndol Forte for pain and another one called Endep for nerve pain. I walked out of the office thinking, 'I'm an actual sick person now.'"

Even though the doctor approved of the Vitex, she asked Jess to put it aside for two months and to take a synthetic progesterone instead. She took it for one month and it caused continual spotting. It also put her into a premenstrual state. Jess described herself during that time as being "lethargic and like this crabby bitch."

After four weeks, Jess was absolutely miserable and consulted her GP. She suggested that they stop the progesterone and go back to the Vitex.

"We had the idea that we needed to boost the progesterone and shorten my cycle so that there wasn't this build up, build up, build up in my uterus. I took the Vitex and my symptoms got better. I went from having a 30-day cycle to a 27-day cycle in two months and on the fourth month, I got pregnant."

It was wonderful news, but it had serious implications on Jess's work situation. At the time, she was working at a vet clinic where her duties included x-rays and assisting with surgery. With radiation and anaesthetic gases suspected of being harmful during pregnancy, Jess was obligated to tell her colleagues immediately to ensure the safety of her baby.

The other nurses were helpful in arranging her tasks to avoid exposure and this allowed Jess to continue working. She was immediately nauseous with morning sickness and it was so severe that she lost a huge amount of weight.

> **"I went down two dress sizes while I was pregnant because I felt so 'ugh' all the time. I have never been so skinny in all my adult life. I was previously a vegetarian for 14 years and when I got pregnant, all I wanted to eat was a Whopper."**

Jess's vegetarianism ended during her pregnancy. She recalls being so nauseous that she often needed to pull over on the side of the highway to vomit. One day at around 11 weeks' gestation, Jess felt so awful that she decided to leave work early. She did not feel that she could drive home safely, so she went to her sister's house nearby. Her sister was also pregnant and when Jess arrived, she was having an antenatal appointment with her midwife.

> **"I was supposed to have my first antenatal appointment with the same midwife the following week. I said to her, 'I'm enormous. I'm in maternity pants already.' And she said, 'Let's have a look.' She palpated my belly and said, 'Are you sure your dates are right because you're palpating like 25 weeks.'"**

The midwife suggested that one of the possibilities might be that she was pregnant with twins. She asked Jess to go to the Women's and Children's Hospital for an ultrasound, so Jess called Simon who was busy and said he would call her back. Jess sat by the phone, getting more and more anxious by the moment. Her mind was racing with the ramifications of twins. If it was true, it meant that her dream of a home birth would be over. She also wondered if that was the reason why she had experienced a lot of pain during the pregnancy. Simon finally called and in tears, Jess explained what had happened. She immediately went to pick him up from work and they drove directly to the hospital.

The midwife phoned ahead so that they were expected. The emergency department ultrasound was incapable of showing enough detail, but it did confirm that she was not carrying twins. They returned the following day when the imaging department was open, and the higher-powered machine showed that Jess had a large fluid mass in her abdomen, a cyst measuring 11 cm in diameter and shaped like a football.

A junior doctor came over to provide the couple with the diagnosis and treatment.

> **"She was quite fearful, obviously, and she said, 'You need to have surgery tomorrow. You'll probably have a miscarriage because that might be the ovary that's maintaining your pregnancy. The cyst could twist and torsion or rupture any moment.' I lost it. I told her, 'It's taken two years to get pregnant!' She went to find a supervisor who calmed everyone down and said, 'I've seen this before. It's not going to torsion or rupture in the next five minutes.'"**

Jess was discharged and filled with anxiety about the safety of her baby. A few weeks later, they returned to meet with the consultant who explained that they only had a one-week window to perform the surgery to deal with the cyst. They would have to operate between week 15 and 16 of gestation. Any earlier and they might affect the ovary making hormones to maintain the pregnancy. Any later and she could go into premature labour.

Wanting some clarification on exactly what would happen, Jess went to her trusted GP who advised that prior to ultrasounds, women would often go into labour only to discover that during pregnancy, a cyst had dropped down and blocked the baby from engaging into the birth canal. When this occurred, delivery would become an emergency situation and the baby would have to be delivered by c-section. The surgery at 15 weeks was a better option because it would be done under controlled conditions. This information combined with the confidence of the surgeon and the reputation of the hospital gave Jess the confidence to proceed with the operation.

> **"On the way to theatre, the surgeon said, 'You might lose your ovary. You might not. Best case scenario, your baby is fine. You keep your ovary and it's all done keyhole. Worst case scenario, you lose your baby, you have no ovary on that side, and you've ended up with a laparotomy*.' It was pretty scary."**

At that point, Jess was committed. It was too late to opt out, so they wheeled her in for surgery. Several hours later, she woke up in recovery.

> **"I've never been in so much pain in my life! Ovaries are like testicles, they're sensitive. I remember lying in recovery, just screaming I was in so much pain. They were running around saying, 'Get the Ketamine*' and because I was a vet nurse, I**

yelled, 'Oh my god, that's horse tranquilliser! I'm not taking that! Don't you know I'm pregnant?'"

Eventually the morphine became effective, but it took 48 hours to get her pain under control. The good news was that the surgery, a keyhole procedure, was a complete success.

Jess was cared for by the high-risk unit until her 20-week scan where it was evident that the baby was doing well. It was ironic that the couple had made the decision not to do any ultrasounds except the 20-week scan. They ended up doing multiple scans and the benefit it provided was peace of mind.

The downgrading of her pregnancy to the low risk category restored Jess's plans for a home birth. She resumed her regular antenatal appointments with her midwife and throughout her pregnancy she kept up with all her natural therapies, making extra visits to her chiropractor.

"I had a lot of pelvic instability during pregnancy. I waddled from about eight weeks and I was sore, going to the chiro all the time."

Much of the pain and imbalance may have been due to the position of the baby. Retrospectively, it was evident that rather than presenting in a symmetrical way, the baby's head was tilted to the side and remained that way all the way to delivery.

At 4am when Jess was at 39 weeks and two days gestation, her waters broke. Knowing that delivery could take anywhere up to a few days, Jess was calm, feeling that the contractions were nothing more dramatic than the Braxton Hicks she had experienced over the past 19 weeks.

By 9am, things ramped up. She called the midwife, her sister and a friend to say birth was imminent. Simon set up the pool in the lounge room, filled it with water and Jess got in.

"It's so great for pain relief because you're floating. The gravity is gone so you don't have all that pressure on your parts. But it probably didn't help things progress at a nice pace either."

Jess spent most of the day in the pool with short contractions that were spaced well apart. The midwife was continually monitoring the baby's heart rate and it was not elevated. At 6pm, Jess got out to go to the toilet and she had a few strong contractions.

"They were painful, but I think that just got the head around the bend. And then he was born. He came out with this big cone head, but off to the side, so he would have had a raging headache!"

Harvey arrived weighing over 4kg. Jess was so grateful that she had been at home because she feels that if she had been in a hospital, she would not have been allowed to push ineffectively for seven hours. Due to his presentation, the medical team would likely have insisted on a c-section or at a minimum, an episiotomy*.

"I did have a small haemorrhage afterwards. Because I didn't eat the whole day, I had nothing left, no energy to push out the placenta. We were sitting on the fence on whether or not I should go to hospital. I just wanted to stay home with my baby. And just as I was about to say that maybe I do need to go, I just turned a corner and I was fine."

Due to the substantial blood loss, Jess was unable to walk without feeling light-headed. This lasted for several days and meant that she was bed-bound, other than crawling to the bathroom and back. Her midwife visited the next day but was unable to offer any postnatal care from then on because her licence was suspended due to issues with a client's birth.

"In hindsight, I should have gone and got some more help, but I didn't."

Aside from coping with her own recovery while caring for a newborn, Jess found that breastfeeding was a challenge. She had cracked nipples and when Harvey was a toddler, a GP told Jess that he had a tongue-tie. The other difficulty was getting their newborn to have a proper sleep period because he would wake up 10 times a night. He was also a noisy breather, something that his parents thought was a cute purring sound.

Harvey is now six years old and he still wakes up once or twice a night, but at least they now know why. When they went to see an ENT* surgeon for a second opinion last year, he asked, "So how's his sleep apnoea?" The previous doctor must have noted the problem but failed to advised Jess. That information explained so much of what they had gone through in his first five years.

The ENT also fitted Harvey with grommets* to deal with his frequent ear infections. Jess expressed to me her frustration at the lack of explanation provided by some doctors and she remains unapologetic for continually seeking clarification.

"I always ask questions. 'What if I don't do that? What's the risk if we don't intervene?' They never give me straight answers."

The couple had always wanted more than one child and it was their plan to have another as soon as possible. After nine months, Jess went back to work in a vet clinic and they also moved away from their community to be closer to the city. She remembers this time in her life as being lonely, away from her network of friends and working in a new job that made her miserable.

Jess decided to focus on having another child. She went back onto her naturopathic supplements, Vitex, Chinese herbs, and acupuncturist treatments. At one particular acupuncture treatment, she saw cards left there by a Maya Abdominal Massage* Therapist. She booked a session, hoping it could help with her fertility. She had also been experiencing increased ovulation pain and was worried that it might be another ovarian cyst.

An ultrasound revealed a five centimetre diameter white clump, indicating that it was not fluid, but likely to be an endometriomas* (endometrial cyst) or a dermoid cyst*. Jess consulted her gynaecologist who predictably recommended surgery.

"I knew I had to get rid of that before I got pregnant because I was not going to have surgery during pregnancy again. That was scary."

Before committing to an operation, Jess decided to see if Maya Abdominal Massage could help with the cyst. The therapist was confident that she could help and proceeded to treat Jess, sending her home with instructions on how to do the massage herself and to apply the castor oil packs to her belly.

"I did that for about six weeks. I had a repeat ultrasound next cycle and it was down to two centimetres. I was like, 'I'll just keep doing my thing.' At the next ultrasound after the following cycle, it was completely gone."

From her previous experience, Jess expected it to take a long time to fall pregnant. When it only took two cycles, it felt like a miracle!

"I thought I was lucky because I naively thought that I'd had my hardship. I'd done that. I just wanted peace. But that's not how it works."

The miscarriage occurred one night when Jess was breastfeeding Harvey. She previously noticed her nipples were sore and sensitive and on a midnight trip to the toilet, she discovered a little blood. She went back to bed, then heard Harvey wake again so she fed him. This time, her nipples were not sore anymore. She woke her husband to tell him she thought she was having a miscarriage. Somehow, they went back to sleep, but when she woke the next time there was more blood.

Because they were living in a new area, Jess had not found a new family GP, so she phoned the nearest one and took the next available appointment.

> **"I told the doctor I was having a miscarriage. She asked me how I knew I was pregnant, suggesting that I was just having a period. She wanted me to go wee on a stick and do a pregnancy test. I ended up passing the products in the toilet at the doctor's. I came back to her with the toilet paper and said, 'This just came out. I had to sort of pull it out.' And she said, 'Oh, okay. You probably don't need that ultrasound,' and into the medical waste it went."**

Simon and Jess were stunned by the lack of empathy from that GP. A month later she needed to see her again for another matter, and the doctor asked her if she had recovered from the miscarriage. Jess said that she had not, to which the doctor swiftly interjected with the words, "I mean physically."

On top of coming to terms with the miscarriage, the young family was also dealing with Simon's mental health. All of the intensity of trying to fall pregnant, the challenge of a new baby and of finding the right treatment added to his depressed state.

> **"There were some months where we didn't even try because of what was going on with his health. So I kept doing all my abdominal massage and castor oil packs."**

About eight months later, Jess conceived again. At almost six weeks, the couple ended up in emergency at their local tertiary maternity hospital because Jess's symptoms had disappeared, and she needed reassurance. The sonographer could not find a heartbeat but told them that it was normal. She also saw what she thought looked like second gestational sac, which meant the possibility of twins. The couple was asked to return in two weeks and at that scan, there was still no heartbeat, but the sonographer said it was normal at six weeks.

Simon and Jess questioned the dates, thinking it was six weeks last time, how can it still be six weeks, two weeks later? The doctor in the emergency department suggested that it was likely that Jess had experienced a missed miscarriage and advised a D & C.

"I've had a miscarriage before, my body can do this. I'll just go off and do it. They weren't keen on that."

Jess left the hospital and continued to do her massage and castor oil packs. Every time she applied a pack, she would see spotting and think, "Here we go." Then it would go away and nothing would happen. She continued to see her naturopath, acupuncturist and Maya Abdominal therapist, and these women provided a beautiful circle of care for Jess.

"I had this space held for me by these women. It was amazing."

At 11 weeks' gestation, Jess finally gave up. That morning, she was wet, as if her waters had broken. She went into hospital and it happened again. The medical staff insisted on starting a medically managed miscarriage which was similar to an induction birth. Jess was required to take medication and stayed overnight. Because labour did not progress, she needed a D & C the next day.

Jess is grateful for the wonderful midwife who handled her hospital care. With only two miscarriages, she did not qualify for the recurrent loss clinic, but because of her history, the midwife arranged for the couple and their baby to be tested.

The results on the genetic testing was that the baby had double the number of every chromosome. When the egg and sperm had come together there had been some glitch and instead of 23 pairs of chromosomes the baby had 46.

"If you have one extra chromosome 21, it gives you Down Syndrome. Imagine having double everything? She was completely incompatible with life."

The couple was told that it was just a freak occurrence and that they should try again after Jess had one period. After a 28-day menstrual cycle, sure enough, the next cycle she was pregnant. It was a joy tempered with worry and that was exacerbated by two early episodes of bleeding.

Jess went to her trusted GP, a doctor who was aware of her miscarriages and understood why she was concerned. He arranged a hCG test to check her levels and provided a referral for a second test the next day so that they could compare levels. It was a Friday, but the doctor offered to call her over the weekend with the results. There was a mix-up with the tests and on Sunday night the doctor called to say he was going to wait for the correct results but that might not be until 11pm.

> **"He rang me and said, 'It's gone up and it looks good. How are you feeling?' I said, 'Terrible. I feel like this is the beginning of the end again.'"**

The GP offered to arrange an ultrasound plus a further hCG blood test the following day to reassure her that the pregnancy was fine.

> **"That helped put my mind at ease for all of about five or six days. My emotions were all over the place. I got excited. Then I told myself not to get excited yet."**

The following weekend, Jess bled again and headed straight into the hospital where she was seen by junior doctor.

> **"He was a young, arrogant twat. He asked me when I had my last period and I told him the date but explained that I didn't ovulate until day 21. Then he argued with me about how I would know that, and I told him it is painful for me, and that I'd checked my cervical mucus and the position of my cervix. He asked, 'How often do you put your fingers up there? I'm going to swab you for infection, that could be the cause of blood loss.' I made a complaint about it because as far as I'm concerned, all he should have done is checked things out, like my baby's heartbeat. He was just disgusting."**

The doctor went on to argue with her about home birth, lecturing her about the dangers of delivering outside the hospital. Jess found herself having to justify herself to someone who had no knowledge of her medical history—the entire consultation was invasive and disrespectful.

Still under the care of the recurrent loss clinic, Jess returned to the hospital at 12 weeks for an ultrasound. It showed that Jess had a subchorionic hematoma*, the likely source of the bleeding.

At the same appointment, they also had a nuchal translucency test. Due to the genetic issues with the last miscarriage, the couple decided it was a good idea and they were relieved to find out that their baby was healthy.

The doctors continued to keep a close eye on her pregnancy with regular scans. At 18 weeks, the baby was positioned in a way that prevented the sonographer from getting pictures of the spine and kidney. Jess ended up returning three times and they still couldn't get clear scans. At every appointment, the doctor would push for a hospital birth and this incomplete ultrasound only added to her case.

It didn't help that the baby's due date was in the middle of one of Adelaide's largest festivals which meant that there would be more traffic and people than usual in the city.

> **"She said, 'If you have to transfer, you're not going to get to hospital on time. What if there are no ambulances available? How will you get through the city at that time?' We had these arguments over and over. I live five kilometres from the hospital. So I just stopped seeing her."**

Even though she felt strongly about her right to choose a home birth, the constant comments did play on her mind.

> **"Because I'd had the two losses, I started to let that affect me mentally. Should I go to hospital? Am I being stupid? But I hate hospitals. I'm not going to labour well in a place that I'm completely fearful of. So we went with the home birth."**

Jess continued her antenatal appointments with a new midwife that she found through her midwifery contacts. She handled all the necessary progressive checks and she was also happy to support Jess during a pregnancy that was both physically and emotionally difficult.

> **"Some days I couldn't feel movement and I was stressed out of my brain. I think I rang my midwife twice and asked her to come and listen to the baby's heartbeat, just to hear it. I probably should have done that more, but I didn't want to be a pest."**

To support her mental health, Jess saw a psychologist, the second one that she had seen regularly since her first miscarriage. She found that the sessions helped her to deal with the extreme anxiety about her pregnancy and her worry about bonding with the baby. This stemmed from the fact that Jess knew that this could be her last baby and she held a lot of guilt about wanting the child to be a girl, as she had with the baby that she had miscarried.

"We didn't find out the sex of the baby, but I nearly did. At 20 weeks I thought, 'It might help me bond with the baby if I find out what sex it is.' And then I thought, 'No, it doesn't matter. I've gone through all this, so it really doesn't.' I think you think that you're protecting yourself by not bonding, just in case something goes wrong, but I don't think it works."

One big difference between her two pregnancies was that this time, she put on weight. Jess confessed that she used food to feel better and "ate her feelings". This was compounded by the way in which Harvey was weaned off breastfeeding.

"I breastfed through the two miscarriages and then about 10 weeks into my second pregnancy, my son turned three. He dropped the day nap and was really only feeding just to go to sleep at night. He'd feed for a minute and then he'd be asleep. Because I was pregnant, my milk dried up. I remember feeling so gutted because I wanted it be his decision."

A month before her due date, Jess started experiencing pre-labour with contractions every two or three days for one or two hours. Aware that second births can occur notoriously fast, her midwife and doula* were both expectant and ready to attend to Jess the moment she called.

Days passed and by 39 weeks and five days, there were still no signs of active labour. That night there was a Festival of Lights event in the city and they decided to attend. As the family packed and got ready to go, Jess went to the toilet where her mucus plug* came out. It was a start, but she had no idea how things would progress, so she grabbed a spare pair of knickers and leggings and waddled around the city looking at the light display.

Nothing happened overnight, and the next morning they took Harvey and their dog for a walk to the park. Still nothing. That afternoon, Jess thought she might as well clean the house.

Tired from the housework, Jess collapsed on the couch. She tried to have a nap but any thoughts of sleep were interrupted by a huge contraction. Her waters broke and the excitement began. Or so they thought. The midwife came over to check on her and everything was fine, but her contractions were irregular and there was no telling when the baby would be born so the midwife went home.

In hindsight, Jess realises that her labour was much more established than she let on. By 8pm, she called her mum, sister, the midwife and the doula and Simon started filling up the pool. The midwife arrived at around

8.30pm and Jess got into the pool. After one strong and painful contraction, she wanted to get out of the pool to go to the toilet, but the midwife stopped her because she could see the baby's head coming out.

> **"On my third contraction the midwife bought her up between my legs. Simon was face to face with me and I still remember his face. I have so many photos from Harvey's birth because it went on for a really long time. And I have about four of this one. It was too fast."**

Violet entered the world in record time weighing 3.95kg. Jess was absolutely thrilled to have her girl, filled with gratitude and the recognition of how much energy she had wasted on feeling guilty about wishing for this exact outcome.

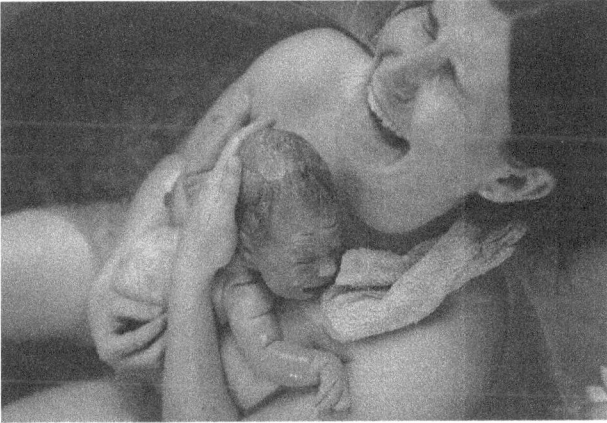

Jess with Violet, moments after birth

The beautiful moment then turned into chaos when Jess's sister pulled up outside the house. The dog started barking and Simon took her out into the front yard so she wouldn't wake Harvey. Simultaneously, Jess was clambering out of the pool because she did not want to birth the placenta in the water.

> **"I had been in the pool for all of 10 minutes. Everyone was anxious about me having another haemorrhage. I got out of the pool and said, 'Oh god, it's coming!' And it just splattered on the floor."**

Her mum, sister and one-year old nephew came in, then the doula arrived and they were all stunned that they had missed the birth. When Jess thinks about how quickly Violet was born, she still wonders how it happened. In relating the two births to me, Jess remarked how interesting it is that each child's personality reflects their arrival.

> **"He's the same as his birth. Everything takes him a really long time. He took a long time to toilet train and a long time to sleep through the night. And she's like a hurricane, a little pocket rocket!"**

It is now two years on and Jess continues the habits she learned throughout her journey. She has struggled with worthiness, making decisions for the good of others rather than prioritising herself. She credits Brené Brown's books for helping her to transform her beliefs. She surrounds herself with like-minded people and practices gratitude as part of her daily life, teaching her children to adopt thankfulness and joy with the family's Joy Jar. Every day at dinner they ask each other, "What made you happy today?" They write the answer on a piece of coloured paper and put it in the jar.

Reflection provides Jess with the perspective to acknowledge how much she has changed her attitudes through things she has learned and the trauma she has experienced.

> **"I used to see drug addicts who had their children taken away from them and my reaction was that they didn't deserve to have children. But now my reaction is, 'What trauma did they go through to make them homeless and drug addicts?'"**

Today, Jess is fulfilling her dream of working with women in a space she is passionate about. She has pursued her original career of massage therapy, specifically Maya Abdominal therapy. During her maternity leave, Jess completed further training to become a qualified Arvigo® Therapist, Womb and Fertility Therapist, Pregnancy Massage and McLoughlin Scar Tissue Release Therapist and she now works exclusively with women, supporting their physical and mental health through her own practice, Earthshine Village.

> **"I listen to their story and I think there's some healing in just having someone listen, someone who knows what it feels like. I just say, 'You didn't deserve it and there is no reason that this happens. It just is. Please ask for what you need and take all the time you need. Everyone heals at different rates.' I don't try and fix them, but I listen and help them with my therapy. So now I've got this purpose."**

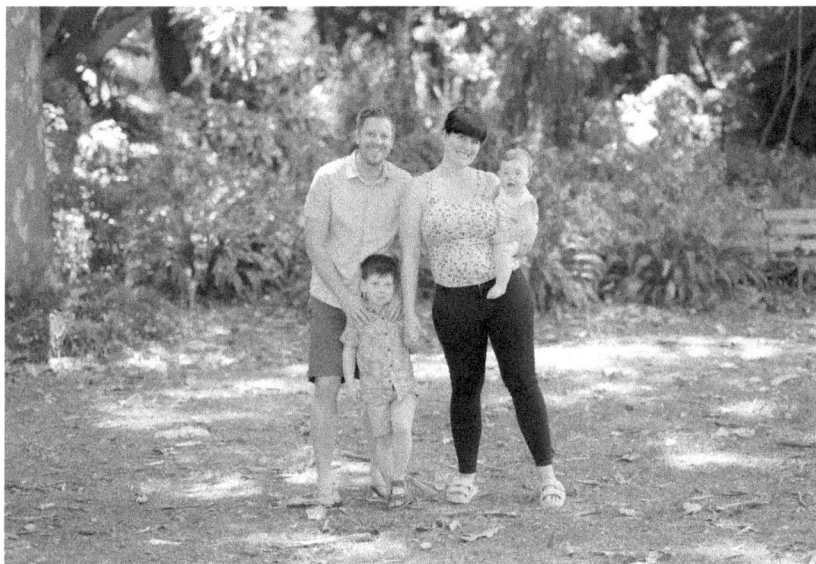

Simon and Jess with Harvey and Violet

"It's finding joy in the small moments. And I think it's even more important in those dark times to just go, 'You know, I had acupuncture treatment today and it was really peaceful and I'm not in pain. If that's all I can ask for today, that's okay. Tomorrow is a new day and we'll see what that brings.'"

18

JEN

- Post-Traumatic Stress Disorder (PTSD)
- Anxiety
- Agoraphobia*
- Assault Survivor
- Twins Emily and Charlie, six years
- Diastasis Recti*
- Miscarriage
- Rainbow baby: Annabelle, four years
- Exploding Head Syndrome*
- Postnatal Depression (PND)
- Postnatal Psychosis*

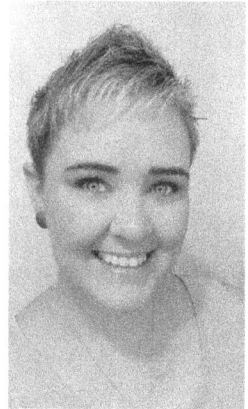

A paramedic at the age of 22, Jen loved being in a job that genuinely helped people. She loved being out and about, but the work presented daily challenges. Jen frequently dealt with abuse from people affected by drugs and alcohol and in the first three years of employment, she was physically assaulted twice and exposed to a situation that caused PTSD.

Jen was only six months into her career when she attended a call to assist an elderly gentleman. Once it was decided that he needed to be taken to hospital, her colleagues went outside to get the stretcher and to better position the ambulance while Jen remained inside the house, packing up their equipment. The man's 42-year-old son was there, and she witnessed a heated argument between him and his wife. His wife stormed out and the man was fuming. With only Jen left in the room, he directed his anger towards her.

"I was cornered between a bed and a sidewall behind me. He stood over me, he was about six foot four, red in the face with veins popping. He was filled with rage and kept yelling profanities and standing over me. And in my head, all I could visualise was him picking me up and throwing me against the concrete wall. With no duress alarm, I was terrified, I thought he was going to kill me."

Fortunately, the man's wife returned and she distracted his attention. This created the opening for Jen to escape out the door. She ran right past the senior paramedic and jumped into the moving ambulance which was being repositioned by her partner. The senior paramedic came over to see what was wrong, giving Jen the opportunity to explain the situation. He replied, "Oh, that's all right. I once had a shotgun to my head."

His response made Jen feel, "Like I had to suck it up. Like it wasn't a big deal because it wasn't a shotgun, was it?" The rest of the day went on as usual and no support was offered. She rationalised that worse things had happened to other people and in the scheme of things, this was probably nothing.

Two weeks later, Jen wheeled a patient into hospital, then went back and sat on the back step of the ambulance. A senior intensive care paramedic saw her and realised that Jen wasn't well. She popped the monitor on Jen and her heart rate was 170.

"She did a specific manoeuvre that brings your heart rate back down, took me into a doctor who prescribed Valium and sent me on my way. These episodes kept happening and it got to the point where I lost the ability to be alone without thinking that I was going to die."

Jen became unable to sleep in a bed by herself, asking her 19-year old brother to stay with her. She would never lock a door behind her in case she needed to get out quickly. She stopped driving her car alone, asking friends, family and work colleagues to transport her to and from work. Jen literally went from being a completely carefree, happy and spontaneous person to being terrified of being alone. She recalls being at the shops and waiting for her mum to do some banking. For a moment, she couldn't see her mum through the crowd of people and she freaking out. This went on for months.

"I was at home having an anxiety attack. I was in tears, in a foetal position. Mum had had enough—she didn't know how to help me anymore. She pulled the employee assistance card out of my wallet, called the number and made an appointment for me to see a psychologist."

Jen was able to work through the events of the past weeks with the psychologist to discover what had caused her current state. Her manager was simultaneously going through her past cases and they discovered that the same man who had traumatised Jen had done the same to another strong female paramedic.

Moving forward from her anxious state was made possible through the continual support of her family, friends, psychologist, medication and a commitment to practicing the tools and strategies she was taught.

"The support from my parents was amazing. My mum would sit up through the night with me when I was in a panic state. She'd try and distract my thoughts, disrupt my thought pattern from my panic mode. She encouraged me to get out of the house and interact with people I felt completely safe with.

Sometimes my best friend and her husband would babysit me overnight. I'd sit at their place in this complete anxiety-struck panic state. And I remember one night my best friend's husband put a Valium in my mouth just to calm me down. He got me some water, I drank it and he carried me to bed to sleep."

The psychologist showed Jen some breathing techniques and exercises. She had a recording that she could listen to and mimic to help her to sleep. At every appointment, she would leave with homework assignments to connect with exactly how her body felt when the attacks occurred. Instead of fighting the panic feeling, she learnt to sit and acknowledge what was happening and to write down exactly what she was thinking and feeling at the time. Jen would take these notes back to the psychologist and they would address these issues and work out new strategies on how to deal with them.

Jen read self-help books and did lots of mindfulness training. She worked hard on herself and it took a year for her to start to live her life freely again.

"If it wasn't for mum picking up that card and making that appointment, I don't think I would have had the conscious

ability to recognise the severity of it. I don't think I would have made that call myself."

Throughout this difficult period, Jen continued to work. Thankfully, she had the support of her manager and colleagues. She remembers her station manager, now retired, who always looked out for her wellbeing. If she noticed Jen was unwell, she would invite her into her office for a rest on the sofa. She would say comforting words and made sure that Jen knew that she was there for her.

"I've always believed that people come in and out of your life for a reason. And if they're not meant to stay, that's okay. Just for that period of time, when I needed her, I didn't have to ask. She'd just say little comforting things like, 'I'm right here. I won't leave you.' She was just beautiful."

After about a year, Jen came off her medication and she was introduced to a guy by friends. They started dating and everything was wonderful at first, but he soon became controlling. He would call her names, forbid her from seeing friends and he would constantly question why she wanted to spend so much time with family. He threw drinking glasses and kicked furniture in her general direction and broke many household items. He frequently stood over her, screaming abuse. He completely isolated her, physically blocking doorways so that she could not leave the house.

This toxic relationship lasted two years and caused Jen to relapse. She finally realised how bad things were and asked a friend to help her pack up and leave.

"My family could see it. And after I'd left, they said, 'We knew. You wouldn't listen to us.' I couldn't see it. So blinded by love, I couldn't see it. He had a way of manipulating me and telling me things that I believed and made me doubt myself. How did this happen? I'm a smart woman. I still think about it. How could he get into my brain like that?"

Shortly after the breakup, Jen decided to purchase a house. She was living there on her own, when fate reconnected her with Ben, the man she had dated when she was 17. Back then, Ben had broken up with Jen to travel overseas. When he returned, it just happened that he was ending a relationship too.

Ben was trying to persuade his ex-girlfriend to move out of his house, but she would not go. One night was particularly bad, and Ben asked Jen if he could stay for a night.

"He came for a night and didn't leave. And five weeks later I was pregnant."

Jen was just 25 at the time and she did not feel ready to be a mum. She was recently single, paying off a house, and wanted to travel before she settled down. She told her mum and could not stop crying because she didn't know what she wanted to do. She told Ben later that evening, again crying, but he was over the moon and this alleviated some of her fears.

The couple had their first scan at 12 weeks and Jen took Ben and her mum along for support. The sonographer whisked the wand across her belly. She moved it again and exclaimed, "There's two in there!"

"I still to this day don't know how I actually felt in that moment. My mum turned around with the biggest grin on her face. I still remember seeing her whole face light up because she was so happy. And Ben had tears in his eyes and a big smile on his face. And I was just bawling my eyes out."

Neither family had a history of twins, and it was certainly not something Jen had ever considered. The shock was significant—just a few months prior she had escaped a bad relationship and was single and free. All her future plans were flipped in an instant. But once she let the news sink in, her mind began to think about her new future and the shock transformed to excitement.

Twin pregnancies can be complicated, so Jen was cared for by the high-risk clinic. She remembers her pregnancy as an amazing experience, a time where she felt energetic and healthy, a perfect example of the pregnancy glow.

"I carried all out the front. I remember putting on a bikini one day and taking a photo of my back in the mirror. I didn't look pregnant, I just looked great. It was fantastic!"

Toward the end of the pregnancy, Jen's doctors advised her to have an elective c-section, explaining that it would be the safest method of delivery for both her and the babies. At the time, she was happy to go with the advice and booked it in, but in hindsight, she believes that it would have been possible to have them vaginally.

At 37 weeks, neither baby was engaged. There was no indication that they were ready to be born, but the c-section still went ahead as scheduled. Jen described it as feeling like the doctors were "rummaging through my handbag" to pull the babies out!

Two healthy baby girls, Emily and Charlie, were welcomed into the world. After delivery, Jen discovered she had diastasis recti, a separation of her abdominal muscles. This caused her to have frequent lower back pain and difficulty standing up for longer than a couple of minutes. This made it physically difficult to care for her babies.

The next challenge was breastfeeding. Jen's milk came in and she was successfully able to feed them both at the same time with the use of a breastfeeding pillow. She has the cutest video of the babies doing synchronised hiccups while feeding!

Things became more difficult when the new family went home. In hindsight, Jen wishes that she had been able to access a lactation consultant, because she had no idea if what she was doing was right.

> **"I had enough milk, but I was lacking in breastfeeding education at the time and I doubted myself. So, I started to top up with formula because they were scrawny, thin babies. I thought my body wasn't addressing the supply and demand. If I had a lactation consultant, she could have explained it to me without me having to question it because you don't always have the questions, but you need the information."**

Jen explained to me that if she had known that top-up feeding can actually inhibit milk production, she would have had a lot less self-doubt. Instead of thinking her poor babies were starving, she would have understood that they were getting what they needed.

> **"All mums have these grey areas in their minds where they don't know if it's right or wrong because no one's shared the information with them in the first place. If breastfeeding is what you want, then work hard for it. If it doesn't work, if you need to go to bottles, that's okay. But make sure to be true to yourself in what you want to do. Don't let other people tell you what you have to do. You don't have to do it."**

After five months of breastfeeding on a strict three-to-five hourly feeding plan, Jen was so fatigued. As the babies grew, breastfeeding both at once was becoming difficult because they would push off the lounge with their feet and play while they were feeding. She started feeding them one at a time but the process with two babies was taking so long that she was barely having 45 minutes in between each feed.

> **"I was physically and emotionally exhausted by the time it took to feed them one at a time. Even with Ben's help, changing**

them in between and burping them, I felt like I was just handing one back and taking the other to do the same thing. It was ridiculous."

This relentless cycle affected Jen's emotional wellbeing. She became anxious about the process of taking them out of the house. The whole prospect of going out in public and needing to feed her babies was overwhelming.

"I just didn't know how I was going to do it. I was still feeding in tandem and I thought, 'I can't go out in public and rip my whole shirt off and feed these babies that I can barely juggle to get up and feed. I needed someone to hand me the child, and then hand me the other one in order to get them on together."

Ben was working long hours and her parents were both working full-time, so none of them were able to assist throughout the day. Jen is forever grateful for her cousin, Alyssa who came over every day for months to help her with the babies. She would arrive early in the morning and stay until Ben arrived home, assisting with bathing and feeding the twins. Jen freely admits that she felt like a "hot mess" and she doesn't know how she could have survived that first year without Alyssa.

Apart from the demanding feeding cycle, Emily and Charlie were healthy babies. By three months of age, they were sleeping through the night. This gave the weary parents the opportunity to finally get some sleep themselves. Jen finally felt able to venture out of the house and the new family settled into a routine that worked really well.

When the girls were around 15 months old, the couple considered having another child.

"So, the thought of making another one was terrifying. Am I going to have two more? What's it going to be? Am I going to be the mum that's got three sets of twins?"

They decided to go for it and Jen fell pregnant immediately. At six weeks, they went in to have their dating scan and confirmed that their calculations were correct. Three weeks later, Jen started spotting. She discovered that she had a subchorionic hematoma and was told not to worry, her body would resolve it.

Jen had arranged for her mum and girlfriend to take care of the twins while she went in to have her scheduled scan. Just before she left home, she had a huge let down of blood.

"I got really anxious and quite panicked, but I kept it together and drove out there. I lay down for the ultrasound, and in the end he said, 'I'm really sorry, there's no heartbeat, I can't find anything.'"

Jen held back her emotions, keeping it together so she could safely drive home, but the moment she saw her mum's face, she broke down and burst into tears. The gestation time was 10 weeks and three days.

"It was so sad because Ben and I had just spent the week deciding what we were going to do to surprise everybody with the pregnancy for Christmas. I had the miscarriage on the twenty-first of November, and my best friend's little one's birthday party was the next day and I still went. I had to go, but I cried all the way there."

When Jen described her emotions during that time, along with the sadness and disappointment, she used the word embarrassment. We discussed the fact that many women who had also experienced miscarriage, felt the same way. Jen believes that these feelings are connected to a woman's fundamental purpose of bearing children.

"Oh my god, I had a miscarriage. We think, 'What's everyone going to think of me? That I can't carry a baby? Why can't we do the most natural thing that we're supposed to do? Why does it go wrong? Why does our body let us down? What have we done wrong to cause it? Why did we cause this to happen?' Yeah, I was embarrassed. It was a really unusual feeling, because I didn't make it happen."

Shortly after Jen arrived home from the ultrasound, her GP phoned to say she had received the results and she asked Jen to come in for an appointment the next morning. The GP gave her a letter to take to the hospital emergency department and, fortunately, a friend's wife was the nurse on duty that day. She asked Jen why she was there, and the tears started flowing. The nurse had experienced miscarriage and IVF herself, so she understood how Jen was feeling. She sat down and explained that she needed to go to the early pregnancy clinic. An appointment was usually required but the nurse called them and arranged for her to go straight over.

After a long wait, they finally saw a midwife who gave Jen the option of going home and letting her body deal with it naturally. It was a Friday, so the midwife recommended that if she had not passed the foetus by Monday, she should return for a D & C.

> **"I was terrified. I didn't want a D & C. I didn't want anybody in there physically removing my baby. I remembered that feeling from the c-section with the twins. I felt that the D & C would be taking my baby from me. I was really grateful for her saying go home. She gave me a script for the pain and a bear to take home. She was a really sweet woman."**

On Saturday night, Jen started having contractions. She did not take any medication and still vividly remembers the immense pain that came with each contraction, something she had not experienced with her previous pregnancy.

Jen laboured in bed, with Ben holding her hand and rubbing her back. After about four hours, it stopped, and she realised that she had actually passed the foetus on one of her trips to the toilet. She had wanted to keep it and plant it and do something special with it, but that didn't happen.

Ben is a quiet man and not one to engage in conflict. He never directly asked how his wife was feeling, but he stayed by her side, refusing to sleep, despite being exhausted after a huge day at work.

> **"He was probably scared of saying the wrong thing and thought it was best to be silent and just be there with me—that was more than enough. There was nothing he could have done to make it any better for me than what he did do."**

Jen realised that the miscarriage was equally difficult for Ben to process and she was wise enough to understand that men experience it and deal with it in a different way to women.

> **"After a few days, I did actually ask him, 'Are you okay? How do you feel about it?' And he shut down. He's like, 'You can't do anything about it. It is what it is.' And that's very much him."**

I asked Jen if she would have approached things differently with Ben. She felt that many men, like Ben, are raised to be tough and strong and to think that showing emotions is weakness. Men go through the excitement of becoming a dad, and therefore feel the loss too. She suggested that men seek out someone who has been through a similar experience, so they could have a man-to-man talk without the emotional investment of the women involved.

Around six months later, the twins were almost two and Jen had not yet had her first cycle after the miscarriage. She had reached the point where she wanted to try to get pregnant and again, she fell instantly.

This time, her excitement was tempered by an equal measure of fear.

> **"Throughout the whole pregnancy, every time I went to the toilet, I was terrified to look down. I didn't want to see blood. Every little cramp I'd get, I was terrified. I would feel this instant panic and dread inside because I didn't want to lose my baby. No matter how many weeks or months along, it was the same."**

Jen found her conscious mind creating dialogue to override her subconscious fears. She would tell herself that there was little chance of it happening again. She'd had perfect twins so this one would be okay.

Rather than sitting around and dwelling on things, Jen kept busy taking care of the girls and working for the New South Wales Ambulance Service. She worked right up until 38 weeks, thinking she would have a couple of weeks to relax and prepare for her baby's arrival.

After her previous experiences, Jen researched her delivery options and set her mind on having a VBAC*, vaginal birth after caesarean. She was in the Maternity Group Practice program and appreciated the availability and contact with her midwife, Christina, throughout her pregnancy. In those last weeks, she walked on the beach daily and took good care of herself in preparation for delivery.

At 40 weeks' gestation, Jen was attending appointments for daily monitoring. Her obstetrician assessed her, saying, "I'll give you a high five if you can have that baby vaginally because it's not engaged. I really don't think it's going to happen for you."

Jen was devastated at the news. For the health of herself and the baby, she eventually came to terms with delivering by caesarean. The morning they were booked in, the couple went to hospital, ready to go. Christina arrived shortly after and right at that moment, Jen became overwhelmed by anxiety about the procedure.

> **"I just completely back-pedalled. I said, 'I don't want to do it. I don't want to be here.' I was so panicked. I wanted to run out the door and hide, I just didn't want to have the c-section. I thought, 'I can't do this.'"**

She begged for more time, for the opportunity to experience real labour. All her hopes and dreams for a VBAC came flooding back.

Christina went to discuss her situation with the obstetrician. She returned shortly after and said, "You owe me." She had managed convinced the doctor to allow Jen one more week. If the baby did not arrive in seven days, she would have to go through with the c-section.

Ben and Jen flew out the door and did everything they could to induce labour naturally. Jen took two beach walks every day. They filled oil burners with clary sage and rosehip oils. They even went online for help and tried all sorts of wacky manoeuvres to get the baby to engage.

A few days later Jen went down to visit Alyssa who lived a 25-minute drive from home. She noticed some contractions and by around 1.00pm, she was getting really uncomfortable and realised that she needed to head back. Jen phoned Ben on the way and arranged for him to look at heading home from work. Once home, Jen contacted her mother who organised for her sister Heather to watch the twins. Jen's contractions were about three minutes apart, lasting for 90 seconds. It was time.

Arriving at the hospital, Jen had a massive contraction and security ran over to her with a wheelchair. She refused, unable to sit because all the pain was in her back. She waddled to the lift, supported by her mum, and it took about 15 contractions to get to the bed. By the time she got there, Christina and the birth photographer were already waiting. Soon after, Ben also arrived.

Christina checked to see what was happening and at that exact moment, Jen's waters broke and exploded all over her!

The mood changed instantaneously because there was meconium in her waters. That put an urgent time frame on the delivery. Jen was in so much pain, unable to sit, stand or lie down. She was on her knees, leaning and rocking.

Using gas to get through the last part, Jen gave a few good pushes and heard the baby's heartbeat on the monitor change. Christina asked her to stop pushing and to breathe through the contraction because the baby's heartbeat was plummeting.

The baby was posterior forehead first, and the umbilical cord was over her shoulder, pinching between Jen's pelvic bones and her shoulder. Every contraction was cutting off the baby's blood supply.

Christina hit the emergency button, then helped her up onto the bed and rolled her onto her side to increase blood flow to the baby.

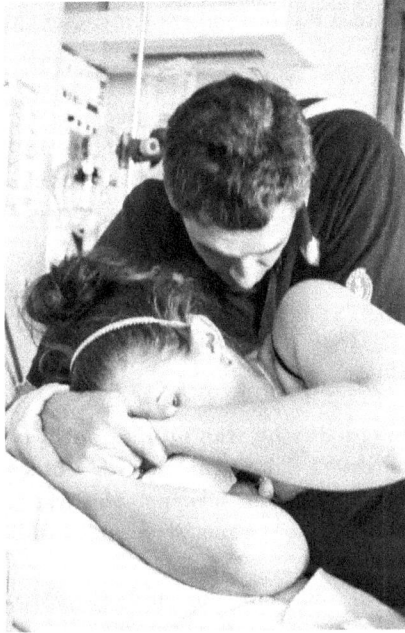

Jen and Ben during labour

The anaesthetist came in and administered an epidural between contractions. The first dose was not effective, so he delivered a second dose. Fourteen medical staff arrived including a paediatrician and the obstetrician.

It was absolute pandemonium. There were nurses everywhere: one inserting an IV, others wiping Jen down with antiseptic wipes in case they had to go to theatre, and another helping Ben get into a gown.

The obstetrician examined Jen and confirmed Christina's assessment, before advising the best course of action as a forceps delivery. This was the one thing Jen had discussed with her midwife as a definite no go. She had read about cases of babies delivered via forceps who were badly hurt with cuts, scarring and brain damage. She would rather have an emergency caesarean than that.

Sensing her concern, the obstetrician pulled up a chair and sat next to her, creating an oasis of calm amidst the chaos. He asked Jen why she had concerns about forceps, and that gave her the opportunity to express her fears. The obstetrician listened intently before replying, "They're not my first choice as an obstetrician, but the baby is too high for a vacuum. How about we get you into theatre and I'll reassess? If anything changes between here and there, I'll just do a straight caesarean. I won't hurt your baby."

"I definitely think that I felt safe because of the way they approached me and considered my thoughts and feelings in the decision-making process. They included me in it, and that doesn't happen all the time, so I feel so lucky that I had that team, that day."

Jen looked at Christina for reassurance, and with her agreement everyone moved into theatre. The obstetrician performed an episiotomy and delivered their daughter.

"Ben said it looked like he was pulling out a tree stump! Out came Annabelle, this 3.95kg bruiser with a black eye and not a mark on her head from the forceps. She was a fat, beautiful baby who looked like she'd gone 20 rounds with Rocky."

Thankfully, Annabelle did not succumb to Meconium Aspiration Syndrome, and her airways were clear. Jen did suffer a postpartum haemorrhage and lost around 800ml of blood. This left her feeling fatigued but otherwise, well.

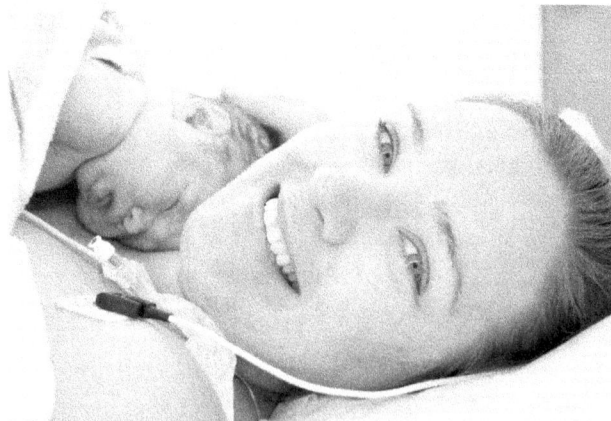

Jen with Annabelle

"It was a traumatic birth, but not psychologically. It was just crazy. Here's me picturing this beautiful, pain-free, drug-free VBAC birth, and it was the complete opposite. And I'm okay with that."

After five days in hospital, Jen went home and was thankful that Annabelle slept well and breastfed beautifully. In fact, the hardest part of bringing the new baby home was not the baby, it was coping with the two-and-a-half year-old twins!

Ben went back to work following his two weeks of paternity leave, and Jen was left to mother the girls and a newborn on her own.

> **"I couldn't cope. I cried so many tears, thinking I was failing those twins by not giving them any attention, not giving them what they needed. They would be mucking up and really naughty and I couldn't deal with that. I couldn't discipline them. And I had Annabelle to tend to as well which takes up a lot of time. I found I was crying constantly, but never in front of anyone."**

Jen internalised her emotions because she felt that she should be able to cope. Adding to these personal feelings of failure, she was also haunted by things that her family had said to her after the twins. Things like, "Oh, you're crazy to have any more babies. You don't need any more. You've already got two, they keep you busy enough."

Despite all this well-meaning advice, the couple had wanted another child, so when Jen really needed help to cope with the three children, she didn't ask.

> **"I was automatically defensive, thinking I shouldn't ask these people for help because they don't respect or agree with what I am doing. I should be able to do it myself because I wanted it."**

With the family on one income, Ben was working long shifts, leaving home at 3am and not returning until 10pm and therefore was unable to offer hands-on support. The situation became progressively worse until the point where Jen felt paranoid. She developed a condition known as exploding head syndrome, hearing loud explosion-like noises just as she was drifting off to sleep.

This was compounded by postpartum psychosis causing Jen to hear voices.

> **"It was hell, it was so scary. I had no control. But I wouldn't share it with anybody. I was embarrassed for myself at that time. I was convinced I was losing the plot. That terrified me. I thought, 'I can't go in a loony bin, I've got these kids to care for and Ben's got to work. Everyone would be so disappointed in me and I couldn't hack that.'"**

Jen was in fear of herself. She was crying all the time and unable to cope with the kids. One day she was sitting on the lounge, holding Annabelle, and the twins were wanting her attention. Jen just sat crying, staring at them.

At that moment, her neighbour, Bren, knocked on the door and Jen just broke down. Seeing how distressed she was, Bren found the twins' shoes and hats and took them out, telling Jen to go next door for a chat with his wife Mel.

"She's so beautiful. I just sat and talked with her and cried and she made me a cup of tea. After five weeks of feeling hopeless, she really helped me, she completely reset me."

Reaching the point of crisis helped Jen realise that she really did need help. She was due for her six-week check-up and as her regular GP was unavailable, another female doctor came in and asked how she felt. This simple question triggered a flood of tears. The GP recognised the signs and asked her to fill out a mental health assessment. Her questionnaire score revealed that Jen needed immediate support and the doctor started her on some medication to assist her to regain her mental balance.

Jen was not sure how she would react to the drugs, so she sensibly went to her mum's place with the girls to take her first dose.

"Mum knew I was a broken mess because she'd gone through all of that with me before. I remember her saying, 'I don't want you to have to do this again, not the medication, but the struggle.' She was so overwhelmed with fear for me, that I wouldn't be okay because she carried me before through all that hell for years."

The medication worked and her mood stabilised. Like her mother, Jen hopes that her girls do not have these issues—her family history shows that all the women on her mother's side, including her mother, have suffered from anxiety, panic attacks and postnatal depression and she believes it is the result of hormonal and genetic links.

The other element that contributed to Jen's recovery was her psychologist, a practitioner who specialises in mindful focus. This, combined with medication to rebalance her brain chemistry, gave Jen the tools to move forward.

"I'm still on the medication, four years later, but weaning myself down. We've got to get rid of the stigma, that being on

some sort of medication is a problem. If the chemicals in your brain aren't balancing, then you need something. If you've hurt your arm, you need something. It's no different."

Ben and Jen's home is filled with gorgeous family photos, a reflection of their strong and happy home. Jen continues to work on herself, taking care of her own wellbeing and this ensures she can be at her best as wife and mother.

Jen has spoken to many other women about their birth experiences. Some women she has met had a wonderful prenatal and birth team, while others tell of regrets and difficulties. These stories, combined with her personal experience, inspired Jen to work in midwifery, and she is currently at university, studying to become a qualified midwife herself.

"My midwife delivered beautiful care. She was awesome and I had such a positive experience, prenatally, intrapartum and postnatally. It made me want other people to feel the same way. I want to give this to other women.'

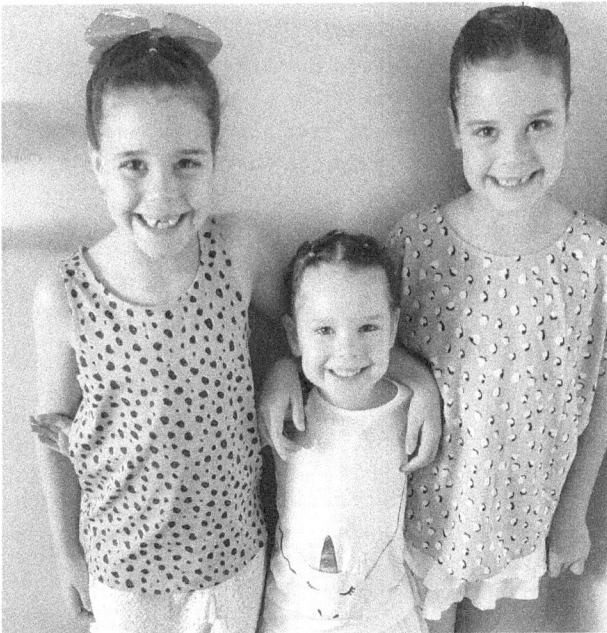

Twins Emily and Charlie with Annabelle

19

FOR PARENTS: HOW TO SURVIVE-REVIVE-THRIVE

Nobody is immune to difficulties in pregnancy and birth. On Good Morning America, singer-songwriter and actress Beyoncé famously shared details of her miscarriages and pre-eclampsia during pregnancy with her twins.

> **"I was in survival mode and did not grasp it all until months later. Today I have a connection to any parent who has been through such an experience," she said. "I learned that all pain and loss is a gift. I needed time to heal, to recover."**

If you are struggling with your own difficulties around pregnancy and birth, know that you are not alone. Your struggles and loss do not diminish you. It is possible to find a way forward and I hope that the stories in this book have helped you to find strength for your own journey. Every person's experience is individual, but perhaps you have been able to relate to someone's story, their physical pain or their emotional anguish.

I have so much love and gratitude for the families who were willing to share their most intimate feelings during stressful and anxious times that for some, lasted for years in their quest for a child. For those who have lost a child, my heart is filled with sadness—you have my utmost respect for the way in which you honour them.

The emotions surrounding pregnancy and birth are complex. For a woman, the very definition of being female is "denoting the sex that can bear offspring or produce eggs." (Oxford Dictionary).

We grow up believing that our bodies will be able to perform the natural function of reproduction because we are equipped with the organs for the task. It is part of our identity and our period serves as a monthly reminder of this role.

When we experience difficulties with fertility, it is unlike any other medical issue we have with our body. If we have problems with any other organs, we go to the doctor and do whatever is required to rectify it. But with fertility, there are so many other concerns and factors that come to bear.

There is the optimal window for healthy pregnancy and as women age, it brings an anxiety about running out of time to conceive. There is the societal pressure of well-meaning friends and family who constantly ask women of a certain age when they will have a baby. And when things don't go to plan, there are the feelings of shame and frustration when our bodies don't perform.

There is no magic wand to make the pain, anger, sadness, worry and devastation disappear. What we can do is to be empathetic and remove all judgement of the choices and actions of other women. We can be supportive of each other and share experiences and knowledge with each other. We can raise awareness about the real and visceral impact of pregnancy and infant loss, dangerously ill newborns and postnatal anxiety and depression.

The wonderful people I have met in the course of writing this book have shared the things that helped them to cope with their trauma and allowed them to move forward. I put them together in the following pages in the hope that they can bring some light to your situation and help you to move through the process of surviving, reviving and thriving.

TAKING CARE OF YOUR BODY

Doctors are Humans

Depending on your individual journey, you may see medical professionals before and during pregnancy and after birth. If your baby is unwell, you may also see other specialists including paediatricians. As you will know from hearing other people's experiences, sometimes we have medical consultations where we feel uncared for or misunderstood. In the same way that we don't connect with everyone we meet, so too it is with medical practitioners. Not every doctor or specialist is the right fit.

So many couples who shared their stories spoke of advice given that was not truly appropriate to their needs. The important thing to remember is that doctors are humans too. Their advice is based on the best of their knowledge and experience.

For some reason we tend to believe that a doctor's diagnosis and advice is irrefutable fact. It is not. Doctors do not have crystal balls to divine the future; they can only provide an opinion based on what they know and the medical history you have shared with them. What a medical professional offers to you is the expected outcome according to their understanding.

The story of Jane is a perfect example of this. She was told by a doctor in no uncertain terms that she would never have children and yet today she is the proud parent of a healthy little girl. If the advice you are given does not sit well with you, do not hesitate to get another opinion to either verify what you have been told, or to provide a different perspective on your situation.

Seek Information

There are many places to look for information. When you research online, check the sources and credibility of the material presented. There are a growing number of organisations who support the specific areas of early miscarriage, stillbirth, infant loss, birth trauma and early parenting. If you are suffering from postnatal anxiety and depression, these support groups can also assist with your emotional and mental health by connecting you to counsellors and psychologists who specialise in these areas. You will find a comprehensive list of support organisations in the back of this book.

Each of these organisations offers a diverse range of support services with many providing written resources, access to peer support, Facebook groups, helplines and counselling. Through your own investigations, you may discover options that you were not made aware of at your medical consultations.

In particular, the organisations that support new mothers offer specialised services that doctors do not have the resources to help with. There is no need to struggle with babies who won't settle or breastfeed. Find local centres and services who can help you with solving these difficulties so you can stress less and be reassured about what you are doing.

If you think that you've found something that applies to you or an option that someone else has tried that could work in your situation, write it down and ask your doctor about whether or not it could work for you.

There is no harm in asking—the worst thing that can happen is that your doctor says, "No," and explains why it won't work for you. Who knows, it could be an option that was not previously considered for a multitude of reasons. If you bring it up, it could open the door to a better outcome.

Talk to Peers

There is nothing better than talking to someone who is experiencing or has experienced what you are going through. Even though their situation may be different to yours, the similarities can offer ideas and solutions that you may not have otherwise discovered.

Jess used a number of therapies to ease her pain during pregnancy including acupuncture. I wish I had thought about this option when I was pregnant as it may have been extremely beneficial. Finding out what works for other people who have been there and done that is a tried and true method of discovering better ways to do things.

Perhaps someone reading Nerida's story will ask for the split bilirubin test for their persistently jaundiced baby and it may very well save their newborn's life. These are the things we can learn from each other when we share our experiences.

Ask Questions

If the doctors explain things in medical jargon that you cannot understand, ask them to clarify what they are saying. Rather than waiting and wondering, ask for information so you can be involved with your care. Remember that it is your body being treated and once born, your baby's wellbeing that is at stake. It is imperative that you fully understand what procedures are being done and why.

When Angus and Nerida were told that their newborn had a life-threatening disease, they were hit with a bucketload of complicated medical terminology associated with her complex diagnosis. They researched what they could online and asked many questions of their medical team in order to understand and come to terms with her prognosis. The couple has cultivated a good relationship with Chloé's doctors, and this contributes to their daughter's excellent care.

Speak Up

Medical staff are not mind readers and many issues occur due to miscommunication. If you don't tell them about further developments in your symptoms, they won't know what you need. Because we are all raised to be polite and to not make a fuss, sometimes we put up with worsening symptoms when we don't need to.

Don't be afraid to speak up about anything that concerns you. Remember the story of Renee who was admitted to hospital for the birth of her first baby. Four days after having the induction gel applied, she still had not given birth. The staff was dealing with 13 unplanned caesareans, so it was incredibly busy in the birthing suites and this was part of the problem. But on reflection, she also believes that the lack of attention was in part due to the fact that she did not "make enough noise to get the help needed."

If the hospital staff are busy, be patient. It is unlikely that they are intentionally ignoring you and more likely that they are dealing with the urgent. Give them time to respond, but don't give up—keep calm and continue to seek their assistance when you need it.

The Right to Choose

The strongest piece of advice from many women was to find the team to best support you through your pregnancy and birth. For some, hiring a doula and a midwife provided the reassurance of individual and personalised care. For others, attending the high-risk clinic on a regular basis was the path to ensure their baby's safety. Some women choose to have their own obstetrician while others decide not to have any scans. There are those who work right up until delivery and others who choose special eating plans.

There is no right or wrong way to be pregnant, deliver a baby, or parent a child. Absolutes do not belong in this arena. When I asked women about their regrets, many of them talked about the perceived pressure to make choices based on what they thought they should do rather than what they wanted to do.

Sometimes there are impossible decisions that must be made. The stories of Sara and Rebecca illustrate how important it is to make the right decision for yourself and your family. You will remember that both women were told at around 20 weeks that their babies had chromosomal abnormalities with chromosome 18. If the babies survived birth, it was unlikely that they would have any quality of life or lifespan.

Rebecca make the choice to terminate the pregnancy and gave birth to Lucas at around 23 weeks while Sara carried Jonathon to term and he lived for 14 hours. Both families experienced immeasurable pain, grief and sadness. Neither choice was better or worse. Each of them made the most informed decision they could and I have the utmost respect for the strength it took to make those choices and live with the outcomes.

You have the right to choose as well as the right to change your mind. Take some time out and let that inner dialogue of "should and should nots" go. Find out what your gut feels is right. Talk to your loved ones and trusted confidants about your fears and concerns. In this way, you can determine what choices are right for your emotional wellbeing, your body and your family. You might still have questions and "what ifs" in your mind, but by pausing to work out what you really want, then instead of feeling like you have been pushed into a decision, it will be your conscious decision.

Be Flexible

Even with the most carefully laid plan, the unexpected can happen so it is imperative to also be flexible. Some of us are planners, others of us prefer to go with the flow. In consultation with your doctor or midwife it is definitely a good idea to have a preferred birthing scenario but to also be ready to move to a contingency plan if things don't happen the way that you hoped.

Think of Kaz's story, the midwife who had her mind set on a home birth. When the time came and her baby was breech after two days in labour, she had to surrender and go to the hospital for her own health and that of her baby.

According to Dr Simon Winder, an obstetrician and gynaecologist who specialises in high-risk obstetrics, early pregnancy, genetic conditions and infertility, he often sees couples who want to stick rigidly to their plan.

"My idea of a good delivery is where I get a well mother and a well baby. If you get to do the route that you want, then that is a bonus, but that should not be your focus. This whole idea of what is natural is all well and good, but death is natural too and that is the harsh reality of it."

"If someone comes in with a list saying, 'I want this,' and things aren't going well, I think the best plan is to be as flexible as possible because the problem with coming in with a really preconceived idea of what you want is that they just don't see the bigger picture, they lose all situational awareness."

Your wellbeing and the safe delivery of your baby are the top priorities so be open to changes. Ask your medical team to explain the situation so you can understand why and what needs to be done.

. . .

Trust your instincts

If you feel that something is wrong, then keep investigating until you get answers. So many women talked to me using words such as, "I instinctively knew something was not right," or "My instincts told me something was wrong." We know our bodies and when things are not as they are supposed to be.

You will remember Katherine's story. When she saw spotting at 10 weeks' gestation, she went straight to the hospital and was told that everything was fine. She went home, feeling that something was definitely wrong. Returning to hospital the next day, Katherine asked for an ultrasound and found out that she had actually miscarried. If she had not followed her instincts, this may not have been discovered until her next doctor's appointment.

The same instinctual feeling made Sally go to the doctor the day after she discovered she was pregnant. When she was diagnosed with an ectopic pregnancy, she required immediate surgery. Sally experienced massive blood loss with internal haemorrhaging and if she had not trusted her instincts, she may not have reached the hospital in time.

Time to Heal

When a woman becomes pregnant, her body is flooded with hormones, geared up for the task of growing a baby. No matter the outcome of your pregnancy, your body has undergone a dramatic change and it will never be exactly the same again.

We all know those incredibly lucky people who can get back in their pre-pregnancy jeans within a few weeks. My sister was one of these women and I remember being green with envy as she easily transitioned to her regular wardrobe within six weeks. Meanwhile, I had gained 12kg during my first pregnancy and felt like a human balloon for months! It took me a year of careful eating and exercise to get that weight off!

Even though my sister appeared to be back to her pre-pregnancy state, her body was as forever changed as mine. After our tummies had expanded so dramatically, why would they spring back to exactly how they were before? If you stretched an elastic band for nine months, it surely would not spring back to its original size.

Many of us put pressure on ourselves to restore our bodies and of course, each of us has a choice to make about how to do this. Whatever you decide, be kind to yourself. Don't set unrealistic expectations that cause anxiety and diminish your self-esteem. Each of us needs time to heal from the physical effects of pregnancy and birth and it is important to give yourself the time and space to heal and to come back to a new normal.

Complementary and Alternative Therapies

There are varying opinions on the efficacy of complementary and alternative therapies. Medical professionals can sometimes be sceptical because there are limited studies and research to support the positive effects. Even though there may not be documented medical benefits, more and more hospitals and medical professionals agree that they provide a positive benefit to a patient's wellbeing.

An example of this is the Chris O'Brien Lifehouse that works alongside the Royal Prince Alfred Hospital and the University of Sydney to improve the quality of life for cancer patients, carers and their families. Patients receive essential treatment including surgery chemotherapy and are offered a range of evidence based complementary therapies to support and restore patients to health. Some of these therapies include acupuncture, exercise physiology, massage, physiotherapy, meditation, reflexology and yoga.

Some people report brilliant outcomes from these types of therapies, while others have not felt the same kind of results. Many people I have met tell me that they were sceptical before they tried and experienced these therapies for themselves. Some therapies were better than others and when they found the ones that worked for them, they often became strong advocates for the therapy.

Here are some of the therapies found to help body and mind during and after pregnancy:

Acupuncture - A treatment that involves inserting fine needles into the skin at specific points with the aim of balancing the flow of energy. It used to cure illness and relieve pain. For people like Adele, acupuncture was instrumental in improving her reproductive system resulting in her much wanted pregnancies.

Massage: One of the oldest healing traditions. It is the practice of kneading or manipulating a person's muscles and soft tissue in order to improve their wellbeing and health. Maya Abdominal Massage Therapy is specifically effective in treating the reproductive organs with specialist practitioners such as Jess who works with women to assist with menstrual wellness, fertility pregnancy and postnatal healing.

Chinese Herbalist: Nearly 3 million Australians visit Traditional Chinese Medicine practitioners annually. Chinese herbs are prescribed to normalise imbalanced energy and are often used in conjunction with acupuncture. Chinese herbal medicines are mainly plant based, but some preparations include minerals or animal products. A practitioner will diagnose a patient and create a particular concoction of herbs accordingly.

Naturopathy - Uses natural remedies to help the body to heal itself. The goal of naturopathic medicine is to treat the whole person—mind, body and spirit. It aims to heal the root causes of an illness, not just stop the symptoms.

Chiropractic - The maintenance of the spinal column and the adjustment of misaligned joints. More than one million chiropractic adjustments are given every day, all over the world. Around 50% of women experience back pain during pregnancy. Chiropractic care is considered safe during pregnancy and it can greatly relieve these symptoms. It is also an effective treatment to restore health and alignment after childbirth.

Osteopathy - Specialises in the treatment of the musculoskeletal system through the manipulation of muscle tissue and bones. In pregnancy, osteopaths can assist with lower back, hip, pelvic and sciatic pain.

Yoga - A mind and body practice with a 5000-year history in ancient Indian philosophy. There are various styles of yoga that combine physical postures, breathing techniques and relaxation. Investigate which style is best for you. You can access yoga classes locally, online and through apps.

Pilates - A low-impact exercise that aims to strengthen muscles while improving postural alignment and flexibility. There are mat classes and also classes that use a specialised piece of equipment called a Pilates reformer.

TAKING CARE OF YOUR MIND:
MENTAL HEALTH AND EMOTIONAL SUPPORT

The transition from person to parent is one that can be researched and studied but until you experience it for yourself, it is impossible to understand the impact it will have on your life.

I spoke to Dr Winder at length about the trends he has observed in the mental health of his patients during his many years of practice. As is mandatory, he uses the Edinburgh Postnatal Depression Scale (EDPS) screening tool to identify women who may benefit from follow-up care.

"Pregnancy is a stressful life event—physically, emotionally and psychologically for a lot of women. About one in four women will go into full-blown postnatal depression. And a

small percentage, about one in a thousand will go on to have a sort of psychotic episode that is brought about by having had a baby. Traditionally people say it is just the hormones of pregnancy. It's not just the hormones, it is a major life changing event. Suddenly there's that realisation that you are no longer just looking after yourself or yourself and your partner, there is now a little person who does not come with a manual."

Dr Winder has extended the EDPS screening to include men.

"About one in 10 men also get some form of postnatal depression and I suspect that it is probably also driven by a lack of sleep. There may be worries about how they are going to support their partner and the baby because they were a two-income family and now they are not. So, there are all those sorts of pressures that are on men, that they are thinking about. But they are not thinking, 'I am going to get postnatal depression'. Very, very occasionally, I will find a dad who scores worse than mum."

"We (men) are not very good at talking about how we feel. We tend to bottle it up. It is sort of seen as a sign of weakness. I remember growing up. If you fell over and were hurt, you were told to get up straight away. I would start bawling and get told to toughen up. It is that kind of attitude."

Dr Winder's findings illustrate how the mental health of both men and women are affected by the transition to parenthood. Realising that there are many others experiencing similar challenges and that there is no shame in asking for help are keys to helping new parents cope with a role that is filled with a multitude of challenges.

When pregnancy does not go to plan and ends in miscarriage, there is an even greater need for mental and emotional support. Dr Winder notes that the impact of miscarriage is different for every individual.

"It is a bit of a spectrum when I am dealing with miscarriage. For some people it is the absolute, most horrible, worst experience in their life. For other people it is like, 'Okay, it is a shitty universe. Let us go again. How soon can we start again?' And everything in between."

"But I will say some women who have had miscarriages or have had terminations for various reasons, even 10 or 20 years down the track, they are still harbouring all the guilt about that. When I am counselling somebody talking about miscarriage, I always say, 'The first question we going to ask ourselves is, why has this happened to me?' Valid question. The next question they ask is usually, 'What did I do to cause this?' And then, when they are finished flogging themselves with that one, it is, 'What did I not do that I should have done, that caused this?'"

"And I just sit there and say to them, 'Nothing and nothing. It is a shitty universe we live in. That is how it rolls. It is not your fault.' And sometimes, I have got to say it two or three times before it actually hits and they finally say, 'Oh, it is not my fault.'"

There is no right or wrong way to feel when you experience pregnancy trauma. Whatever you feel is real and does not need to be justified. The path to healing yourself is yours to choose. What I want you to know is that there is help available to you at every stage. I invite you to investigate the following avenues that men and women have used to heal their pain and move forward.

You are Not Alone

When you experience trauma, it will inevitably affect your life in some way. No one can know exactly how you feel because you and your situation are unique, but there are those who have been through similar experiences. Even though no one in your circle of family and friends can truly understand how you feel, hearing stories of those who have walked a similar path can help you to feel less isolated and alone. Stories such as the ones you have read in this book present people from all walks of life who have felt the same pain, frustration and sadness. Each of them has tackled their challenges differently and perhaps you can relate to the way they have moved their life onwards.

The subjects dealt with in this book are only now starting to be discussed openly and honestly. Even a decade ago, subjects such as miscarriage and fertility were rarely shared but rather hidden away as if there was some shame in not being able to conceive successfully. Even today, when the subject is raised in conversation, women who reveal their past issues around pregnancy and birth admit that they never felt able to talk about it before.

One of the ways we can all help women and families to feel safe in sharing their pregnancy and birth trauma is to increase awareness about these issues and to change the long-held social etiquette of not talking about these things. When one in four pregnancies end in loss, six in every 1000 babies is stillbirth and one in every 10 babies a premature birth*, pregnancy and birth issues are affecting a large proportion of the population and the emotional trauma caused by these losses and sick newborns must be addressed to assure the mental health of families.

Talking about it and sharing experiences is the first step to feeling that you are not alone. You will be surprised by the number of people who, once you tell them about what has happened to you, will disclose that they have been affected themselves or by a loved one who has gone through a similar experience. The shared information can build supportive bonds and form new friendships.

Friends and Family

When you are going through a traumatic time, close friends and family may want to do everything they can to support you. Some may run around trying to do practical tasks for you, others may give you well-meaning advice. As wonderful as this may sound, in reality, they might be driving you crazy.

The important thing here is to work out what you need to feel supported. As time passes, this may change, so the vital ingredient is communication. Be thankful and grateful for the efforts that people are making and make sure they know you appreciate their good intentions. But if they are helping out in ways that are not sitting well with you, gently redirect them to something that would be acceptable. When they feel unable to make you feel better, if you ask them to do some practical task such as provide a home-cooked meal or pick up some groceries, then that saves you from needing to do it and it also allows them the satisfaction of feeling helpful.

Remember the story of Renee and Tim who had both sets of their parents with them at the hospital every day while Zac was in the NICU. There were times when the couple needed some space to be alone and it was important to communicate this to their respective parents in a way that expressed their appreciation but still gave them some time out.

Some friends and family may have difficulty processing your situation and you may not hear from them. This does not necessarily mean that they do not care. Perhaps your trauma has reignited a past pain for them and being with you in that moment might be too confronting. There could be many other reasons why they feel unable to engage so don't write them off.

On the topic of friends and family, we need to address the 12-week rule. There is much discussion about this unspoken societal construct that dictates that we should not tell anyone about our pregnancy within the first 12 weeks in case something happens. There are no actual clinical guidelines as to when you should or should not announce a pregnancy.

The secrecy around early pregnancy means that couples who experience miscarriage often grieve in private, weighed down with feelings of guilt and failure. We have not told friends and family that we were pregnant, so how can we now say that we have miscarried? At the very time when support is most needed, we fail to share our emotions and seek help. We all want to appear happy and successful—perfect Instagram photos and videos of the happy families of friends and celebrities subconsciously create more pressure on us to hide ourselves away or to put on a brave face.

You will remember the story of Tahyna who was absolutely devastated by her miscarriage. At dinner with her flatmates that evening, she was visibly upset but felt unable to explain her loss because they had not yet shared the news of their pregnancy.

When discussing the 12-week rule with Dr Winder, he acknowledged the current debate over when to tell people they are pregnant. He shared two cases that demonstrated it has to come down to a personal choice.

The first case involved a woman who had an early foetal death in utero. She shared her pregnancy news immediately with her mother, sister and two daughters and they were all excited to come together with her to the ultrasound.

> **"I was scanning and had to say, 'I am sorry, this baby is not going further. It is no longer here.' That generated a whole heap of grief and upset. I later asked her, 'We talk about the 12-week rule. What would you do in hindsight?' I was really interested in her perspective and she said, 'I would not tell anybody again.'"**

The second case involved a situation with a family that had strict religious beliefs. Dr Winder identified a foetal anomaly.

> **"That opens up a whole can of worms for some people. The responses from some people outside their immediate support group were really quite judgemental about termination. But I can guarantee that if those very same people were in their shoes, they would come to exactly the same decision. Not telling people avoids that scenario. But telling people allows**

people to talk about it and console each other. I guess it's horses for courses. It is not one size fits all."

If you are deciding what is best for you, seek all the information and assurance that you need to make your decision about when you feel that the timing is right for you.

Peer Support

From my discussions with many families, one of the most helpful things they did was to seek the support of others who had endured similar experiences. They did this through in a variety of ways, including online groups, face-to-face groups and social media groups.

Peer support groups offer many benefits. The first thing most people noted was that they felt immediately secure amongst a group of people who knew exactly what they were talking about. They didn't have to explain themselves or feel self-conscious about what they said. It was an instant mutual understanding.

The groups offer a place to share information and to ask questions that friends and family cannot understand. They are a safe place to find out first-hand knowledge of helpful ideas and resources. This nurturing environment is one that can also carry you through new pregnancy issues.

Women tend to be natural sharers, but as noted by Dr Winder, men tend to bottle things up, rather than sharing their feelings for fear of appearing weak. Peer groups connect men to other men who have been through similar experiences and this provides a safe space for them to open up and have frank man-to-man discussions.

If you or your partner are having difficulty in expressing your feelings or processing your emotions, then a peer group can facilitate a helpful dialogue.

Peer groups can be found through support organisation such as those listed in this book. You can also search groups on social media to find the best fit for you.

Professional Support

If you are struggling, it is vitally important to seek medical help. So many of us adhere to the 'soldier on' philosophy, suffering through our illnesses and thinking that they will eventually go away. When it comes to mental health and in particular, postnatal depression, new mums can feel that their sadness will pass and that they are just tired from the sleep deprivation that comes with a newborn.

There are so many myths around the validity of this condition that stop women seeking treatment. Thinking such as, "It must not be PND because it didn't start straight after birth," or "I'm so blessed to have a healthy baby, I have no right to be depressed," or "I'm a strong person, I'll be fine," may or may not be true. A new baby means changed routines, extra responsibilities and tasks. Our nurturing side kicks in and we think about taking care of everyone else first before sparing a thought for ourselves, so perhaps when we are going through this period of our lives, we are not the best judge of how we are tracking.

There is absolutely no harm in seeking help from health professionals. If you are having difficulties settling your baby or with breastfeeding, there are wonderful organisations who offer individual support to assist you to master the right techniques. Just because we are born able to nurture and feed a baby doesn't mean that it is easy. Apparently motherhood is supposed to come to us naturally and there might be some women who take to the role like a duck to water, but for most of is, it is like starting a new job type—you feel like you want to check with someone experienced to ask, "Am I doing this right?"

Feeling out of our depth can heighten our anxiety and depression. If you have any concern whatsoever that you are not coping, or if you have an inkling that you just don't feel right, then ask for help. You can start with your GP who can check your overall physical and mental health. Your doctor can then refer you to specialists to advise on particular issues, including professionals to deal with your mental health.

Your doctor may refer you to a psychiatrist, a specialist who deals with your mental health and will assess if you require medication. In the story of Yvette, you will recall that she was diagnosed with postnatal depression. By the time she sought help, she was in a desperate place and the psychiatrist prescribed medication to help her to cope. She also started regular psychology sessions to process and deal with her trauma.

One of the most vulnerable times is pregnancy after loss. The joy of being pregnant can be tinged with anxiety, worry and sadness. Amanda described how she was stuck in a state of grief following the stillbirth of Eva while she was pregnant with Lillian. It was her midwife who helped her to get her mind out of the past and into the present to connect with the baby she was growing. Amanda realised she needed professional help and her psychologist helped her to work through her emotions to create a loving bond with Lillian.

No matter what you are feeling, please do not judge yourself or downplay your emotions and situation. Go to your doctor and ask for help. The best-case scenario is that you discover that you are coping well. The even better outcome is that if you need medical help, you have made the first step and will get what you need to get back on the path to recovery.

Counselling Support

Psychology, therapy or "shrink" sessions—these are some of the terms use to describe counselling, something that some still view as necessary only for self-indulgent celebrities or people with serious mental illnesses. I beg to differ. Personally, I have had regular counselling for years and it is one of the main reasons I have been able to survive, revive and thrive.

Many of the people in this book also cite counselling as a key factor in their recovery. A confidential meeting with a professionally trained counsellor who has no emotional stake in your situation offers a totally safe place to speak openly without any fear of repercussions or hurt feelings. Sometimes people tell me that they were able to find a friend or family member to confide in. That is a wonderful thing, but because they are a part of your life, you are still inhibited by your care and love for that person. You do not have to worry about hurting a counsellor's feelings, or to stress over concern that your words may affect your friendship. They are not part of your regular life, so you can free yourself to be honest and open with them and, more importantly, yourself. Through this process, you can truly work on restoring your mental and emotional health.

Finding a counsellor can sometimes be challenging. I have had people say to me that they have tried therapy, but it didn't work for them. Once I delve further, I usually find that they only went once, to one psychologist and because they did not connect with that person, they decided that the entire profession did not work!

As I have moved to different places and lived all over the world, I have left trusted counsellors and have needed to seek new ones. I have been referred to some that I felt did not understand me at all. Sometimes I would give them the benefit of the doubt and do a couple of sessions before realising that we were not a good fit and that I needed to move on.

In the same way that not everyone you meet is going to be your best friend, so it is with counsellors. You may need to see a few different ones to find the right one. I don't know how many you may need to see before you connect with someone who you believe can help you. All I ask you to do is to keep searching until you find them. Ask for referrals, contact support organisations and find that valued professional confidante who can provide the help you need.

Information and Resources

An internet search brings a plethora of information on whatever subject you wish to learn about. When you add in social media sources, there are many different voices sharing their opinion as fact. As you seek knowledge, look for credible sources from reputable support organisations. You can find many of these organisations listed in this book.

Opinions and ideas are wonderful but not all of them may work for you. Before trying something that is new, it is always a good idea to talk to your GP, midwife or obstetrician to discuss your options.

Good Habits

There are many things you can do to help yourself heal from any trauma. I have tried all of these things personally as have the many people I have interviewed. These are all practices you can implement to calm your mind, body and spirit.

Mindfulness - This is the practice of being present. It is so easy to let our minds get caught up with memories of the past and the emotions that those thoughts evoke. Similarly, our minds can fill with worry about the future and the possible worst-case scenarios.

By bringing your mind and full attention to what you are experiencing in this present moment, without judgement, simply acknowledging and accepting what is, can help steady your mood and take you away from the past and the future because in your present moment, they do not exist.

Living in a mindful way does not mean that stress and difficulties are eliminated, but what it does help us do is to become aware of our unpleasant thoughts and emotions and this allows us to be more conscious about how we handle them in the moment.

Meditation - Your mind is like a muscle in your body—if you use certain parts of it, those areas become strong. Meditation is a technique to train and cultivate our minds in order to increase our happiness, focus, compassion and wellness.

The mind is normally active, generating a continuous flow of thoughts, sensations and emotions. Meditation does not try to stop your thoughts, but rather, offers techniques to let them go. It is about resting the mind in a natural, non-judgemental awareness.

When you are meditating, the most important thing to know is that it is not about becoming the perfect meditator. You may choose a meditation where you are focussing on your breath. What if you mind wanders? That is perfectly normal. It probably will. The exercise comes when you acknowledge and accept that your mind has strayed onto a thought and then you gently bring it back into the focus.

It is that action that is the exercise, that makes your mind strong. Meditating consistently is like working your muscles regularly. It is the process that brings the benefits. Your goal is not meditation perfection, but regular meditation practice.

There are many different types of meditation. Some are guided, some include mantras, others use music. You can find books on the subject and there are also a huge range of apps available. What type will be the best fit for you? The best way to find out is to try different ones and see what suits you.

Journaling - There is something both therapeutic and tangible about writing things down. A personal journal can be a private place to write down whatever you experience and feel without fear or filter. Let your thoughts flow freely onto the page. I can type much faster than I can write, particularly if it needs to be legible, but I still put pen to paper for my journal.

There is something visceral about the process and I imagine the act of handwriting as unburdening my mind and allowing the tangle of thoughts to move through my hand and onto the paper in any order. When your worries and feelings are on paper, it moves them to a more objective place where you can see them rather than leaving them hidden away and causing havoc as they roam wherever they choose in your mind.

Writing down positive results and uplifting connections and experiences will help to reinforce the good that is coming into your life. You might have heard about the benefits of keeping a gratitude journal, writing down something you are grateful for each day. When you remind yourself of the good things you already have, it shifts your mind from sadness.

The other positive benefit in writing down your thoughts is that it activates another part of your brain. There have been many studies done on memory and comprehension and educators believe that hearing and reading information brings knowledge into our minds to process. We think about these new ideas and can formulate our views.

But it is only when we verbalise or write these thoughts down in our own words, that the magic happens. We activate different parts of the brain that cause us to evaluate those thoughts and process them before we write them down. In this way, journaling can help you to process the overwhelm of thoughts, worries and emotions that can swamp you throughout your journey.

Helping Others - As you will have discovered from reading the stories in this book, many women have used their personal experience as the impetus to help others who are struggling with the same traumas. My personal experiences are the reason why I have started on my mission to offer light, hope and help to those suffering from trauma.

It is the same reason that sparked Samantha to create Pink Elephants and Melinda to start Made with Love—Murrum. Now these women are helping to ease the journey of others dealing with similar situations.

Helping and learning about what others have been through certainly provides perspective on our own lives and can help to change our outlook. There are many ways to give back and obviously your level of involvement is up to you. Perhaps you can offer support and care to a friend who has experienced pregnancy difficulties. You could offer your friendship as a peer mentor through a support network, group or online group. From my experience and that of others who have been mentors, the joy and fulfilment in helping someone else provides immense satisfaction to both the giver and receiver.

PARTNERS

There is much evidence to show that men and women grieve differently. If your partner is experiencing difficulties in pregnancy or loss, she may be distressed or upset and worried about what's to come. She may turn inwards and feel that she does not want to talk, or she may want to express everything she is feeling.

What can you do? Take your cues from her—if she wants to talk, be there and listen. This is no time to offer solutions or platitudes. Don't say things like, "It wasn't meant to be," or "At least we already have kids," or "It's not the end of the world," We often say these types of things when we don't know what else to say. They are general sayings that just roll off the tongue and show a lack of thought and understanding of her personal situation.

What she needs is for you to listen without judgement or suggestion and to know you hear her. There is no time limit on how long she may be sad or grieve and even though you might wish she would get over it, saying that or acting impatient or intolerant will have the opposite effect. Give her the time she needs, a listening ear anytime she wants to talk, even if she says the same things she has said before.

If she withdraws, ensure that she knows that you are there for her and that you love her. Be there when she needs you and show that you mean it by being reliable and dependable with the smallest task. Show some initiative and help out with the household chores such as cleaning and washing without expecting acknowledgement or appreciation. She might not say it, but she will notice and be grateful that you have taken care of these things.

If you feel that she is not coping well and needs help, there is absolutely no shame in seeking help. Offer to facilitate an appointment with your GP to check on her physical and mental wellbeing. Connect with a local support group and go together to network with others who have first-hand experience on moving forward from similar trauma.

As a partner, you also may be hurting. Men can find themselves in the strange position of experiencing a new kind of pain and grief, with no resources to cope with these unexpected emotions. Society is changing but many men have been raised to bottle-up their feelings, that showing emotion is displaying weakness. Men are meant to be tough and self-sufficient. Sharing thoughts on coping with difficulties is too exposing.

Partners need emotional support and sometimes the best way to do this is to speak to other partners of women who have experienced pregnancy difficulties and loss. According to Dr Elwood David Watson in *The Good Men Project*, reaching out to another man can offer a fresh perspective on a situation.

> **"Men can be more vulnerable with other men than the women in their lives. Men can serve as valuable mentors for one another. The fact is that there are times when people of the same gender can provide advice in ways that others cannot."**

For men, processing your own emotions is as crucial as supporting your partner. In the same way that it is essential to put on your own oxygen mask before helping others if you are on a plane, so too is it vital to ensure your own mental wellbeing in order to best support your partner.

There is no magic formula or instant fix to healing from trauma. Recovery is a process of moving with and through the pain until it gradually lessens. Think of yourself as a tree, caught in a gale force wind. It is ripping through your branches, placing stress on every part of your body, blowing leaves from your branching limbs and shredding bark from your trunk.

If you withdraw and hide from the world, severing your roots, your connections to family and friends, your whole tree might topple over.

Without a strong root system of support, you are not getting the nutrients you need to heal, and this causes your branches to become brittle and to break.

But if you stay connected to support, if you bend with the wind and allow it to pass through, you will be irrevocably changed, but you will remain. To bend, you need to nurture yourself with choices that make you physically and mentally healthy so that your branches are always green, growing and flexible.

Through self-care, acceptance and supportive relationships, you will be able to bend without breaking. You will survive and from there, you can rebuild yourself, reviving your dreams so that you can become a better self, growing and thriving with a new resilience and hope for the future.

20

FOR FRIENDS AND FAMILY: HOW TO PROVIDE
REAL SUPPORT AND UNDERSTANDING

How do you help a friend or family member through pregnancy or infant loss? You may not have known she was pregnant. You may have heard of her miscarriage through someone else. Should you address the subject or wait for her to say something? What are some tangible ways you can offer practical support? What is the best way to give emotional support?

If you have experienced pregnancy or infant loss personally, you will remember the impact of these events in your own lives and can call on your own bank of knowledge to know the best ways to help others. Something important to remember is that not everyone feels the same way as you do—they have their own set of individual circumstances that have contributed to the way they feel about their own situation.

A study conducted by Dr Tom Bourne and his associates in late 2019 revealed an insightful look into the mental health of women who experience early miscarriage loss. Published in the American Journal of Obstetrics and Gynecology, the study found that 29% of women had symptoms of PTSD one month after their loss, and after nine months, 18% reported that the symptoms persisted. Almost a quarter of those women surveyed had moderate to severe anxiety and 11% experienced moderate to severe depression.

"We feel that many people have not understood that for many women, miscarriage or ectopic pregnancy will be the most traumatic event that has happened in their lives up to that point," concluded Dr Bourne.

For those who have not experienced pregnancy, infant loss and ill newborns, it is hard to imagine how people facing this heartbreak must feel. Even though we are not in their shoes, studies like Dr Bourne's can help us to gain some sort of understanding as to the immediate and long-term effect of this type of trauma.

Open communication and conversation around the pregnancy and loss space has progressed somewhat over the past couple of decades, but there is still a long way to go. Women of all ages tell me about the shame and guilt that they feel over pregnancy loss, even when they intellectually know that it is not their fault. This is on top of dealing with the grief and sadness for the loss.

As friends and family, what can we do to support women and men during this incredibly challenging time? There are some wonderful resources available from reputable organisations, many of which are listed in this book. In particular, the downloadable resources created by The Pink Elephants Support Network are brilliant. They address ways to deal with your emotional wellbeing and answer many of the burning questions for those seeking answers.

Knowing what to say to a friend or family member who has experienced trauma and loss is perhaps the most difficult social interaction there is. How do you say the right thing? We feel so much anxiety because we don't want to say the wrong thing and cause more hurt to someone who is already traumatised.

Even though we may know the details of what has occurred, this does not tell us how the events have affected our loved one. They could be feeling sad, shocked, numb, jealous, guilty, empty, lonely, angry, resentful, scared —do not assume to know how they feel because no two people are alike.

I asked the people I interviewed about what family and friends said and did that was and was not helpful. Many of their responses were similar so I put them together here as tips to help you provide sincere and meaningful support.

What to Say

There is no doubt that no matter what you say, your intentions are good. Words have different connotations, however slight, to different people and your choice of words said to soothe and calm your friend or loved one may be perceived as insensitive. Here is a list of some words that women experiencing pregnancy and infant loss have found to be inappropriate:

"I know just how you feel."

"It's a blessing in disguise."

"You've got to read/watch/listen to this. That's what I did when it happened to me."

"You can always have another one."

"It must be God's will."

"Just as well it happened now rather than later."

"It wasn't meant to be."

"At least you know you can get pregnant."

"It wasn't a real baby yet."

"Lots of people have miscarriages, they're common."

"There was obviously something wrong with it."

"You wouldn't want to have a disabled child."

"Aren't you lucky that you already have children."

There are no words that can make her feel better or that will take her pain away. The best thing you can do is to acknowledge her loss. Most women I talked to agreed that a short expression of your understanding is all that is needed. Simple words such as:

"I'm sorry for your loss."

"I'm sorry you are going through this"

"I know how much this meant to you."

"I'm so sorry this happened."

"I'm here for you."

According to Samantha Payne, Co-Founder of The Pink Elephants Miscarriage Support Network:

> **"Never say, 'At least.' There is no 'At least' with loss and miscarriage grief. Pregnancy loss is grief. We need to validate a woman."**

Samantha believes that the key to meaningful support is to listen, empathise and validate women.

Pink Elephants Ambassador, Tahyna McManus lends her support to these principles:

"Don't dismiss it. Really take the time to listen and to let her talk about it."

The most important thing you can do is not to talk, but to listen. If she does not want to talk, make sure she knows that you are there when she is ready to do so. Take the time to check in with a message to let her know you are thinking of her.

What to Do

Is there anything you can do to ease your friend or family member's pain? Take your cues from her. Offer your support and assistance and let her know you are available to help with practical tasks. Here are some suggestions:

1. Offer your time, your presence and a listening ear
2. Drop in a home-cooked meal
3. Help with transport to and from activities for other children
4. Provide transport to medical appointments
5. Do errands and grocery shopping
6. Provide babysitting for other children

She may not respond to your messages or offers and may feel withdrawn. If you are worried about her state of mind, speak to her partner and encourage her to seek professional advice. Give her space but check in at intervals to see if her needs have changed and to make sure she knows of your genuine care and unwavering support.

The most important thing you can do is to be there. You personally may or may not agree with her choices. You may think she is overreacting or emotionless. Whatever you think you would do is irrelevant when you are supporting someone through trauma. Leave your criticism and judgements at home because they have no place here.

To provide meaningful support, you need to offer comfort, and real empathy. It's about showing respect and genuine understanding, assuring them of your unconditional love.

21

SUPPORT ORGANISATIONS

AUSTRALIA AND NEW ZEALAND

Action to Improve Maternity
Supporting families and preventing tragedies. Counselling via telephone, email or in person.
Web: www.aim.org.nz

Angel Casts
Creators of tangible keepsakes for bereaved parents in the form of ink prints and hand and feet stone casts.
Web: www.angelcasts.co.nz

Australasian Birth Trauma Association (ABTA)
Established in 2016 to support women and their families who are suffering postnatally from physical and/or psychological trauma resulting from the birth process as well as the education and support for the range of health professionals who work with prenatal and postnatal women.
Web: www.birthtrauma.org.au

Australian Breastfeeding Association
Resources to help you with breastfeeding and early motherhood. Access to breastfeeding education classes, counselling, the helpline and local support groups.
Web: www.breastfeeding.asn.au

Australian Multiple Birth Association
To enable positive health outcomes, awareness and equality for multiple birth families through advocacy, education and community.
Web: www.amba.org.au

Australian Psychological Society
Pregnancy support counselling. Information and access to Medicare-funded psychological services under the Pregnancy Support Counselling Medicare Scheme.
Web: www.physchology.org.au

The Babes Project
Helping families thrive by creating safe spaces and innovative avenues for vulnerable women to access vital perinatal support.
Web: www.thebabesproject.com.au

Baby Center
The world's number one digital parenting resource with information and support that reaches more than 100 million people monthly.
Web: www.babycenter.com.au

Babyology
An Australian parenting site that provides a supportive and trusted community for over one million parents and parents-to-be.
Web: www.babyology.com.au

Bears of Hope
Providing leading support and exceptional care for families who experience the loss of their baby with support packs, support groups, workshops and counselling.
Web: www.bearsofhope.org.au

Better Health Victoria
Pregnancy support and resources for pregnant women in Victoria.
Web: www.betterhealth.vic.gov.au/health/servicesandsupport/having-a-baby-in-Victoria

Beyond Blue
Advice and support for new and expectant parents, covering everything from bonding with your baby to anxiety and depression.
Web: www.beyondblue.org.au/pregnancy-and-new-parents

Black Dog Institute
A not-for-profit facility for diagnosis, treatment and prevention of mood

disorders such as depression anxiety and bipolar disorder.
Web: www.blackdoginstitute.org.au

Birthline Pregnancy Support

Counselling services, maternal assistance and no-cost resources to help you
with crisis accommodation, education programs, pregnancy mentoring
and antenatal care.
Phone: 1300 655 156
Web: www.birthline.org.au

Bounty

A parenting community with articles, product guides, expert advice,
product reviews and bounty bags.
Web: www.bountyparents.com.au

Brave Foundation

Support for parents to ensure they are connected to help and educational
opportunities in their local communities.
Web: www.bravefoundation.org.au

Bub Hub

The Bub Hub is dedicated to helping you find the information and local
services you need to bring calm and success to your fertility, pregnancy and
parenting journey.
Web: www.bubhub.com.au

The Bump

Expert pregnancy and parenting advice. Includes pregnancy symptoms
directory and connection to forums.
Web: www.thebump.com

Catholic Care (Catholic Family Services)

Helping Sydney families with relationships, parenting, aging, disabilities,
addictions and mental health concerns.
Web: www.catholiccare.org

Centacare (Catholic Community Services)

Pregnancy support including accommodation and counselling.
Web: www.centacare.org.au

The Centre for Perinatal Health and Parenting

Services to support you physically and mentally through pregnancy, birth,
and parenting.
Web: www.perinatalhealth.com.au

Centre of Perinatal Excellence (COPE)
Providing support for the emotional challenges of becoming a parent.
Devoted to reducing the impacts of emotional and mental health problems
in the prenatal and postnatal periods.
Web: www.cope.org.au

Continence Foundation of Australia
Helpline, app and pregnancy guide to assist with incontinence, prolapse,
pelvic floor and sexuality.
Web: www.continence.org.au/pages/pregnancy.html

Earth Shine Village
Treatments for menstrual wellness, fertility support, pregnancy nurturing
and postnatal healing. Arvigo® Therapy, Womb and Fertility Massage
Therapy and Pregnancy Massage by Jess.
Web: www.earthshinevillage.com.au

Essential Baby
Articles, information and resources on fertility, pregnancy, birth and baby
development.
Web: www.essentialbaby.com.au

Focus on the Family
Provides a wide range of programs and resources to support and help
families thrive at every stage of life.
Web: www.families.org.au

Feel the Magic
A not-for-profit organisation creating a world where children who are
experiencing grief are supported to reach their full potential.
Web: www.feelthemagic.org.au

Genesis Pregnancy Support
Counselling, resources, emotional support, education and encouragement
for young mums and mums-to-be.
Web: www.genesispregnancysupport.org.au

Gidget Foundation Australia
A not for profit organisation supporting the emotional wellbeing of
expectant and new parents to ensure that those in need receive timely,
appropriate and supportive care.
Web: www.gidgetfoundation.org.au

Grieve Out Loud
Helping families find their way back to life after pregnancy and infant loss.
Web: www.grieveoutloud.org

Having a Baby in Canberra
Brought to you by the Women's Centre for Health Matters (WCHM), a community-based non-profit organisation which works in the ACT and surrounding region. Information and resources to assist if you are having a baby in the ACT.
Web: www.havingababyincanberra.org.au

Health Direct
A government-funded service providing quality, approved health information and advice.
Web: www.healthdirect.gov.au

Hearts and Minds
Miscarriage support for families in Auckland, New Zealand. Empathy, emotional and psychological peer support.
Web: www.heartsandminds.org.nz

A Heartbreaking Choice
Supports families who have made the heartbreaking choice to terminate a much-wanted pregnancy.
Web: www.aheartbreakingchoice.com

Heartfelt Photography
A volunteer organisation of professional photographers from all over Australia and New Zealand dedicated to the gift of photographic memories to families that have experienced stillbirths, premature births or have children with serious and terminal illnesses.
Phone: 1800 583 768 (Australia)
Phone: 0800 583 768 (New Zealand)
Web: www.heartfelt.org.au

Homebirth Australia
The peak national body for homebirth in Australia. A group of consumers, midwives, and related health professionals committed to ensuring the survival of homebirth as a birth option for Australian women.
Web: www.homebirthaustralia.org

Honestly
Good, clean fun skincare. Traditional aromatherapy with scientific research to create natural skincare that is safe and really works. Crafted by

hand in Australia, Honestly products combine essential oils and minimal ingredients for maximum benefit.
Web: www.honestlystore.com.au

Hope House
A caring and compassionate support team for women, their partners and families when experiencing distress or hardship as a result of an unplanned pregnancy or pregnancy loss.
Web: www.hopehouse.com.au

Hyperemesis Gravidarum Australia
Supporting women suffering from nausea and vomiting in pregnancy (NVP) and hyperemesis gravidarum (HG).
Web: www.hyperemesisaustralia.org.au

Jean Hailes
Delivering the latest scientific and medical evidence to create positive change for women's health. Includes everything from fertility and pregnancy to mental health and more.
Web: www.jeanhailes.org.au

Karitane
Providing accessible, evidence-based services that support families to parent confidently. Information and resources for parents' wellbeing and the care of their new baby.
Web: www.karitane.com.au

Kiddipedia
Top tips, recipes and expert advice. Parenting blogs for every parent to achieve their life goals and to nurture their children.
Web: www.kiddipedia.com.au

Kids First
Educational family and support services to help children and families overcome trauma.
Web: www.kidsfirstaustralia.org.au

Kidspot
Information and advice to help mums and dads through every stage from pregnancy to parenting teens.
Web: www.kidspot.com.au

Kiwi Families
Website, email, bulletin-board, phone and pamphlet support and
information for New Zealanders.
Web: www.kiwifamilies.co.nz

Life's Little Treasures Foundation
Support and friendship for families of premature or sick babies. The
Foundation's services are available in hospitals (neonatal and special care
units) and in the community when families come home.
Web: www.lifeslittletreasures.org.au

The Lost Ones
A New Zealand site dedicated to the ones lost through miscarriage,
stillbirth or SIDS and to the ones they leave behind.
Web: www.thelostones.co.nz

Made With Love—Murrum
Provides a little comfort to families experiencing the loss of a baby.
Provides packs to families, funeral homes and hospitals with clothes,
blankets and keepsakes.
Web: www.facebook.com/helpingcreatealittlecomfort/

Mamamia
A media company with the purpose of making a better place for women
and girls. An online lifestyle hub for women's news and opinions across
many subjects.
Web: www.mamamia.com.au

Maternity Choices
A national consumer advocacy organisation committed to the
advancement of best-practice maternity care for all Australian families.
Web: www.maternitychoices.org.au

Memories of an Angel
A social enterprise to raise awareness for pregnancy and infant loss
through the distribution of keepsakes to bereaved families.
Web: www.memoriesofanangel.com.au

Miracle Babies Foundation
Supporters of premature and sick newborns, their families and the
hospitals that care for them.
Web: www.miraclebabies.org.au

Miscarriage Support
Information and support to women and families throughout New Zealand
who grieve for the loss of their babies.
Web: www.miscarriagesupport.org.nz

Mummylink Young Mums Support Groups
A friendship group connecting young, isolated, lonely and unsupported
mums aged 25 and younger who have a child under three years old.
Phone:08 8352 4044
Email: genesispregnancysupport@msn.com

Mum Central
Premier lifestyle hub for women, parenting, lifestyle, beauty, fashion, food
and travel.
Web: www.mumcentral.com.au

Mum's Grapevine
A parenting website for new mums. Handy tips and tricks to make your
parenting life better plus the best Australian and New Zealand baby
products.
Web: www.mumsgrapevine.com.au

MumSpace
Support for the mental health and emotional wellbeing of pregnant
women, new mums and their families.
Web: www.mumspace.com.au

National Association for Loss and Grief (NSW)
A leading provider of support and education for communities, families and
individuals impacted by loss, grief and trauma.
Web: www.nalag.org.au

National Diabetes Services Scheme (NDSS)
Pregnancy support and resources to support women with diabetes before,
during and after pregnancy.
Web: www.ndss.com.au

National Pregnancy Support Helpline
Free 24/7 helpline for women, their partners and families throughout
Australia. Telephone support for pregnant women and new parents who
have a baby up to 12 months of age.
Phone:1800 882 436

National Women's Health
Comprehensive information on fertility, pregnancy and birth presented by the Auckland District Health Board in New Zealand.
Web: www.nationalwomenshealth.adhb.govt.nz

The Neonatal Trust
Supporting families of premature or sick full-term babies as they make their journey through neonatal care, the transition home and onwards.
Web: www.neonataltrust.org.nz

Newborn Baby
Articles and information on every aspect of pregnancy and birth from conception to newborn.
Web: www.newbornbaby.com.au

New Zealand College of Midwives
Information on pregnancy, preparing for baby, labour and birth and postnatal care.
Web: www.midwife.org.nz

Ngala
A community-based organisation that has been helping Western Australian families for more than 130 years, working to enhance the wellbeing and development of children and young adults.
Web: www.ngala.com.au

Northern Territory Pregnancy, Birthing and Child Health
Services and resources for pregnant women and parents in the Northern Territory.
Web: www.ntgov.au/pregnancy-birthing-and-child-health

Office of Women's Health (ONH)
With a vision to help all women and girls achieve the best possible health, this website offers extensive information on all aspects of reproductive health.
Web: www.womenshealth.gov

Parenting Ideas
Resources for parents to help people successfully raise confident, happy and resilient kids.
Web: www.parentingideas.com.au

Parentline
Free counselling and support for parents in Queensland and the Northern Territory.
Web: www.parentline.com.au

Parents-Guide Illawarra
Online information regarding local services and events relevant to parents of babies, toddlers and school-aged children right up to tweens and teens in the Illawarra.
Web:www.parents-guide.com.au

Parent-Infant Research Institute (PIRI)
Information to help you understand postnatal depression and anxiety.
Web: www.piri.org.au

The Perinatal Loss Centre
Resources for anyone affected by pregnancy or infant loss.
Web: www.theperinatallosscentre.com.au

Pillars of Strength
Helping men in their grief loss after losing a child at birth or at any time, through creating new communities and networks and events for bereaved dads.
Web: www.pillarsofstrength.com.au

Pink Elephants Support Network
Miscarriage support with trusted information, emotional support resources and peer support program.
Web: www.miscarriagesupport.org.au

Post and Antenatal Depression Association (PANDA)
Support for individuals and families to recover from perinatal anxiety and depression.
Web:www.panda.org.au

Pregnancy Birth & Baby
Advice on pregnancy and parenting. Supporting parents on the journey from pregnancy to preschool.
Web: www.pregnancybirthbaby.org

Pregnancy, Birth and Baby Helpline
Free, confidential information and counselling for women, their partners and families relating to issues of conception, pregnancy, birthing and postnatal care.

Web: www1.health.gov.au/internet/main/publishing.nsf/Content/phd-pregnancy-helpline

Pregnancy Birth & Beyond (PBB)

A public health information website providing an extensive source of well-known and up-to-date information and support throughout pregnancy, birth and parenting.
Web: www.pregnancy.com.au

Pregnancy Counselling Link (PCL)

A community agency staffed by professional counsellors. Supports women on issues affecting them in the area of pregnancy, parenting, relationships, navigating life changes, fertility issues and loss and grief. Also supports partners and other family members.
Phone: 1800 777 690
Web: www.pcl.org.au

Pregnancy Counselling Services

Counselling services for New Zealanders involved with a worrying pregnancy. Face-to-face and phone support offered.
Web: www.pregnancycounselling.org.nz

Pregnancy Help Australia

Connects you with a judgement free community who can answer your questions and give you the support and encouragement you need if you are challenged by pregnancy or pregnancy loss. Offers 24/7 helpline, face to face counselling and text chat. Free of charge and confidential.
Helpline: 1300 139 313
Web: www.pregnancyhelpaustralia.org.au

Pregnancy Loss Australia

Support and guidance for miscarriage.
Web: www.pregnancylossaustralia.org.au

Queensland Pregnancy and Family Planning

Information and resources for pregnant and new mums in Queensland.
Web: www.qld.gov.au/health/children/pregnancy

Radiant

A social enterprise of Relationships Australia NSW to help you find a mental health professional that suits you. Guides you in asking the right questions when looking for professional help and connects you to the right professional.
Web: www.myradiant.com.au

Raising Children
Provides parenting videos, articles and apps backed by Australian experts.
Advice on pregnancy and children from newborn to adults.
Web: www.raisingchildren.net.au

Red Nose Grief and Loss
Formerly SIDS and Kids, this organisation has over 40 years' experience
supporting grieving individuals and families after the death of a child.
Offers a comprehensive support library and 24/7 professional help.
Web: www.rednosegriefandloss.org.au

Relationships NSW
Offers resources and counselling to talk about any family issues.
Web: www.relationshipsnsw.org.au/support-services

Remembrance Photography
New Zealand photography of stillborn and terminally ill babies to help
parents remember.
Web: www.remembrancephotography.org

Remember Me – Illawarra Baby and Child Loss Community
A support group for parents who have experienced pregnancy loss, still
birth and neonatal death.
Web:www.facebook.com/remembermeillawarra

Sands
A volunteer-based organisation providing individualised care from one
bereaved parent to another, giving support and hope for the future,
following the death of a baby. Provides miscarriage, still-birth and
newborn death support.
Web: Australia: www.sands.org.au
New Zealand: www.sands.org.nz

Services Australia
Payments and services to help when you have a baby.
Web: www.servicesaustralia.gov.au/individuals/subjects/having-baby

Starting Blocks
Information and tips for early childhood education and care.
Web: www.startingblocks.gov.au

Stillbirth Foundation
Dedicated to research and education to prevent stillbirth.
Web: www.stillbirthfoundation.com.au

Tresillian

Australia's largest early parenting service offering professional advice, education and guidance to families with a baby, toddler or pre-schooler. Tresillian has helped generations of parents over the last 100 years providing reassurance and support with settling babies, sleep difficulties, feeding, multiple babies, toddler behaviour and parental emotional and psychological wellbeing.

Phone: 1300 272 736

Web: www.tresillian.org.au

Twins Research Australia

Twin-specific support and services, including psychologist and mental health advice, telephone services, online community groups and more.

Web: www.twins.org.au

Twin Loss NZ

Supporting families who experience twin loss.

Web: www.twinlossnz.wordpress.com

VeryWell Family

A modern resource that offers a realistic and friendly approach to pregnancy and parenting. More than 5,000 pieces of content created and refined over the past 20 plus years.

Web: www.verywellfamily.com

Young Pregnant and Parenting Network

A mission to help pregnant young women make free and informed choices about their future. Helping young parents to build great futures for themselves and their children.

Web: www.youngpregnantandparenting.org.au

UNITED KINGDOM AND EUROPE

Action on Postpartum Psychosis (APP)

A peer support network helping women and families affected by postpartum psychosis feel understood, supported and less isolated.

Web: www.app-network.org

All About Fertility

Articles, webinars and videos created by doctors, scientists and consultants in the fertility field. Includes a support forum for men.

Web: www.all-about-fertility.com

A Lust for Life
Multi-award winning Irish mental health charity based in Ireland with
content, resources and tools to empower people to cope with life's
challenges and improve mental health.
Web: www.alustforlife.com

Antenatal Results and Choices (ARC)
To provide parents with information and support through antenatal testing
and its consequences and to help them make choices based on their
individual circumstances.
Web: www.arc-uk.org

Association for Improvements in Maternity Services (AIMS)
Providing information and support to women and their families to achieve
the birth that they want through a helpline and sharing information to
pregnant people and health carers.
Web: www.aims.org.uk

Association for Postnatal Illness
Offers support and information for women suffering with postnatal illness
with a network of volunteers who have themselves been affected.
Web: www.apni.org

Best Beginnings
Helping vulnerable families in the UK. Creators of the award-winning
Baby Buddy App, an interactive pregnancy and parenting guide.
Web: www.bestbeginnings.org.uk

Bliss
A vision to provide every baby born premature or sick in the UK with the
best chance of survival and quality of life.
Web: www.bliss.org.uk

Birth Companions
Supporting vulnerable and disadvantaged pregnant women through
pregnancy and birth.
Web: www.birthcompanions.org.uk

The Birth Trauma Association (BTA)
A charity that supports women who have suffered a traumatic birth
experience.
Web: www.birthtraumaassociation.org.uk

British Infertility Counselling Association (BICA)
A place to find a specialist infertility counsellor.
Web: www.bica.net

Chana
Supports couples in the Jewish community who may feel isolated and need
medical information to help them deal with the challenge of infertility.
Web: www.chana.org.uk

Child Bereavement UK
Supports families when a baby or child of any age dies or is dying, or when
a child is facing bereavement.
Web: www.childbereavementuk.org

The Child Death Helpline
Provides support to anyone affected by the death of a child of any age
from pre-birth to adult, under any circumstances, however recent or
long ago.
Web: www.childdeathhelpline.org.uk

Childline
Information and helpline for anything related to children.
Web: www.childline.org.uk

The Compassionate Friends
Understanding, support and comfort to bereaved siblings and parents after
the death of a child in Ireland.
Web: www.tcf.org.uk

Counselling Directory
A directory to find a local counsellor to fit your needs in the UK.
Web: www.counselling-directory.org.uk

Doula UK
Comprehensive information on doulas and how they can support women
through pregnancy, birth and the postnatal period. Access to more than
700 doulas in the UK, Ireland and the Channel Islands.
Web: www.doula.org.uk

Endometriosis UK
Reliable information and support for women affected by endometriosis.
Web: www.endometriosis-uk.org

The Ectopic Pregnancy Trust
Supporting people who have experienced an early pregnancy complication and the health care professionals who care for them.
Web: www.ectopic.org.uk

Emma's Diary
Pregnancy app with gift packs, vouchers, deals and discounts.
Web: www.emmasdiary.co.uk

European Foundation for the care of Newborn Infants (EFCNI)
Dedicated to improving the situation of mothers and newborn infants in Europe. Includes preconception and maternal care, treatment and care of children, follow-up and continuing care of pre-term infants and ill newborns.
Web: www.efcni.org

Family Lives
Advice and support for every stage of your child from pregnancy to teens. Connect to other parents via their online forum or call their confidential helpline.
Web: www.familylives.org.uk

Fertility Friends
A community of members at every stage of their journey from infertility, adoption, parenting after infertility and moving on.
Web: www.fertilityfriends.co.uk

Fertility Network UK
A national charity for anyone who has ever experienced fertility problems.
Web: www.fertilitynetworkuk.org

Good Shepherd
Child and family services for pregnant women and new parents.
Web: www.goodshepherdstl.org

House of Light
Support and counselling for antenatal and postnatal depression and anxiety. Helpline, therapists and support for dads.
Web: www.pndsupport.co.uk

Kicks Count
A pregnancy information guide for expectant mums and dads focussing on baby movement monitoring and a range of support options.
Web: www.kickscount.org.au

Life Charity
Help for pregnancy-related problems. Call, text and messaging services.
Web: www.lifecharity.org.uk

March of Dimes
Supporting mothers throughout their pregnancy. Tools and resources to
assist conception, pregnancy, birth and postnatal care.
Web: www.marchofdimes.org

Maternity Action
Committed to ending inequality and improving the health and wellbeing
of pregnant women, partners and young children from conception
through to the child's early years.
Web: www.maternityaction.org.uk

The Miscarriage Association
The knowledge to help those affected by miscarriage.
Web: www.miscarriageassociation.org.uk

Miscarriage Support
Providing counselling and support services to women and couples of
Scotland who have suffered miscarriage, stillbirth or neonatal loss.
Web: www.miscarriagesupport.org.uk

Mother to Baby
Friendly, expert information about medication and more during pregnancy
and breastfeeding.
Web: www.mothertobaby.org

The Multiple Births Foundation
A national and international authority on multiple births. Employs
healthcare professionals dedicated to supporting multiple birth families
and educating and advising professionals about their special needs.
Web: www.multiplebirths.org.uk

My Baby Manual
Your expert companion on the health, wellbeing and upbringing of your
child before, during and after pregnancy.
Web: www.mybabymanual.co.uk

National Health Service (NHS)
Your pregnancy and baby guide. Discover everything you need to know
about pregnancy, labour and birth and your newborn baby.
Web: www.nhs.uk/conditions/pregnancy-and-birth/

New Parent Support (NCT)
Focussed on providing information, support and connection for parents-to-be and the first 1,000 days of a newborn's life.
Web: www.nct.org.uk

Pandas Foundation
A support group network for men whose wives or partners are suffering from prenatal or postnatal depression.
Web: www.pandasfoundation.org.uk

Parents 1st
A space to find, connect and collaborate with parents, expectant parents, practitioners and volunteers in Essex.
Web: www.parents1st.org.uk

Pelvic Partnership
Supporting women with pregnancy related pelvic girdle pain (PGP). Enabling women to access the right treatment.
Web: www.pelvicpartnership.org.uk

Positive Birth Movement
A global network of antenatal groups. Connecting pregnant women together to share stories, expertise and positivity about birth.
Web: www.positivebirthmovement.org

Pregnancy and Parents Centre
A friendly and welcoming not-for-profit organisation that works with parents-to-be and families in Edinburgh.
Web: www.pregnancyandparents.org.uk

Pregnancy Sickness Support
Information and resources for women with hyperemesis gravidarum.
Web: www.pregnancysicknesssupport.org.uk

Sands
Stillbirth & neonatal death charity working to reduce the number of babies dying and to improve care and support for anyone affected by the death of a baby.
Web: www.sands.org.uk

Tiny Tickers
Improving the early detection and care of babies with serious heart conditions.
Web: www.tinytickers.org

Tommy's
Information and support to empower parents during pregnancy. Evidence-based, expert and user-led information to help expectant parents in understanding what they can do to support a safe and healthy pregnancy.
Web: www.tommys.org

Turn2Us
Assistance to couples expecting a child with benefits, grants or other financial support.
Web: www.turn.2.us.org.uk

Twins Trust
Support and resources for multiple births from pregnancy onwards. Information and community forum.
Web: www.twinstrust.org

UK Government
Information about maternity and paternity leave, registering births, childcare, schools and education, fostering, adoption and surrogacy.
Web: www.gov.uk/browse/childcare-parenting/pregnancy-birth

Verity
A self-help group for women with polycystic ovary syndrome (PCOS). Established to share the truth and improve the lives of women living with PCOS.
Web: www.verity-pcos.orgb.uk

Winston's Wish
Practical services and guidance for bereaved families.
Web: www.winstonswish.org.uk

USA AND CANADA

Abigail's Hope
Blessing families through pregnancy and infant loss.
Web: www.abigailshope.net

A Heartbreaking Choice
Support for those who have terminated a much-wanted pregnancy.
Web: www.aheartbreakingchoice.com

American Pregnancy Association
Resources and helpline for everything from fertility to pregnancy wellness.
Web: www.americanpregnancy.org

Angel Names Association
A non-profit organisation that eases the financial burden imposed by stillbirth. Services for families enduring the trauma of stillbirth.
Web: www.angelnames.org

Angel Whispers Baby Loss Support Program
A non-denominational service for parents who have lost a baby shortly after birth, or during pregnancy, through miscarriage, molar or ectopic pregnancy or stillbirth.
Web: www.angelwhipsers.ca

Association for Pelvic Organ Prolapse Support (APOPS)
A non-profit advocacy agency with global arms, founded in September 2010 to generate awareness of pelvic organ prolapse (POP), to provide support and guidance to women navigating the physical, emotional, social, sexual, fitness and employment quality of life impact of POP.
Web: www.pelvicorganprolapsesupport.org

Babycenter
Answers, tips and information to guide you on the pregnancy journey.
Web: www.babycenter.ca

Bereaved Parents USA
A safe place where grieving parents can connect, share stories and find what they need to rebuild their lives.
Web: www.bereavedparentsusa.org

Birthright International
Based in Canada, Birthright is a safe place to get the information and friendly support to create the right birth plan for each person's pregnancy.
Web: www.birthright.org

Birthwaves
A non-profit organisation that provides doula services to families to experience pregnancy and infant losses.
Web: www.birthwaves.org

Centre for Grief & Healing
Fostering hope and healing for people grieving the loss of a loved one. Peer support and resources.
Web: www.bereavedfamilies.ca

Centre for Reproductive Loss
Professional support services to support the healing of the mind, body and spirit through a holistic approach.
Web: www.crl-rho.org

Childbirth Connection
Information, tools and resources to become an active member of your maternity care team.
Web: www.childbirthconnection.org

Faces of Loss, Faces of Hope
Putting a face on miscarriage, stillbirth and infant loss. Share stories with others who may be looking for reassurance that they are not alone.
Web: www.facesofloss.com

Family Education
Content on everything from choosing baby names, pregnancy, babies and parenting needs to help parents to make the most informed decisions possible.
Web: www.familyeducation.com

First Candle
Committed to ending Sudden Infant Death Syndrome (SIDS) and other sleep-related infant deaths while providing bereavement support to families who have experienced a loss.
Web: www.firstcandle.org

Government of Canada
Pregnancy and baby resources including nutrition, maternity and parental leave, security and benefits.
Web: www.canada.ca

Hand
Helping parents, their families and healthcare providers to cope with the loss of a baby before, during or after birth.
Web: www.handonline.org

Healthy Children
Site powered by the American Academy of Paediatrics. Offers English and Spanish information on a wide range of topics including child development, nutrition, immunisations, mental health and more.
Web: www.healthychildren.org

H.E.A.R.T.S.
Baby loss support program helping empty arms recover through sharing. Compassionate care for grieving Families.
Web: www.heartsbabyloss.ca

Hope Xchange
Shining light on pregnancy loss and grief. Resources to help those coping with miscarriage, stillbirth or infant death.
Web: www.hopexchange.com

International Stillbirth Alliance
Connecting people around the world to prevent stillbirth and newborn death and supporting affected families. A membership organisation uniting bereaved parents and other family members, health professionals and researches to drive global change for the prevention of stillbirth and neonatal death.
Web: www.stillbirthalliance.org

Infants Remembered in Silence (IRIS)
Dedicated to offering support, education and resources to parents, families and friends and professionals on the death of a child in early pregnancy or after birth.
Web: www.irisremembers.com

KellyMom
A website developed to provide evidence-based information on breastfeeding and parenting.
Web: www.kellymom.com

Korie and Kacie
A mission to assist families who have experienced child loss in practical ways including medical bills and funeral funeral arrangements, living expenses, care packages and access to online support groups.
Web: www.korieandkacie.org

Miss Foundation
A community of compassion and hope for grieving families. Providing counselling, advocacy, research and education services to families experiencing the death of a child.
Web: www.missfoundation.org

The Mothers Program
Resources, information and apps for Canadian women before and during pregnancy and after birth.
Web: www.themothersprogram.ca

Multiple Births Canada
A community of families, educators, researchers and health professionals in Canada with a personal or professional interested in the well-being of multiple birth children and those who care for them.
Web: www.multiplebirths.ca

My Miscarriage Matters
A web-based community offering support to the survivors of miscarriage, stillbirth and early infant loss. Connection to peers for tailored guidance.
Web: www.mymiscarriagematters.org

Nationalshare
A community for anyone who experiences the tragic death of a baby. For parents, grandparents, siblings, family and the healthcare professionals who care for grieving families.
Web: www.nationalshare.org

Now I Lay Me Down to Sleep (NILMDTS)
Offering families experiencing the death of a baby the healing power of remembrance. Volunteer photographers provide the free gift of professional portraiture.
Web: www.nowilaymedowntosleep.org

October 15
A site created by bereaved parents. An event directory to showcase the fantastic initiatives that happen every year across Canada to support bereaved families and remember their babies who died.
Web: www.october15.ca

Open to Hope
Resources, stories and community for those who have lost a child.
Web: www.opentohope.com

Orphan Parents
Helping parents experiencing perinatal grief to get through the difficult ordeal. A French language site based in Quebec.
Web: www.parentsorphelins.org

Our Little Angels in Paradise
An online, French-language discussion forum for parents who have lost a child. Offers access to additional French-language resources.
Web: www.nospetitsangesauparadis.com

PANDAS Foundation
Advising and supporting parents and their networks affected by perinatal mental illness. Free helpline, email support and Facebook groups.
Web: www.pandasfoundation.org.uk

Parents
Created to help mums and dads raise happy and healthy kids.
Web: www.parents.com

Parents Canada
Find out everything you need to know about expecting a baby and beyond.
Web: www.parentscanada.com

Postpartum Support International (PSI)
Support, education, advocacy and research for people affected by depression and anxiety during pregnancy and after birth.
Web:www.postpartum.net

Pregnancy After Loss Support (PALS)
Online support groups and in-person meet-ups to support you through trying to conceive, pregnancy and parenting after loss.
Web: www.pregnancyafterlosssupport.org

Pregnancy and Infant Loss Network
Dedicated to improving bereavement care and providing support to families who have suffered the loss of pregnancy or the death of their baby/babies.
Web: www.pailnetwork.sunnybrook.ca

Pregnancy After Loss Support (PALS)
Non-profit organisation and community support resource for women experiencing the confusing and conflicting emotions of grief mixed with joy during the journey through pregnancy after loss.
Web: www.pregnancyafterlosssupport.org

Pregnancy Loss Support Program (PLSP)
Free counselling and support for parents who have experienced miscarriage, stillbirth, newborn death or termination for foetal anomalies as well as women who are pregnant following a loss.
Web: www.pregnancyloss.org

Project Sweet Peas
Empowering and supporting families of fragile infants. Inspiring hope through remembrance for those affected by pregnancy and infant loss.
Web: www.projectsweetpeas.com

Remembering Our Babies
Support, education and awareness for those who are suffering or may know someone who has suffered a miscarriage, an ectopic pregnancy, a stillbirth or the loss of an infant.
Web: www.october15.com

Return to Zero: H.O.P.E
A community of bereaved families and their health providers who are transforming the culture of pregnancy and infant loss through awareness, education and support.
Web: www.rtzhope.org

Sidelines
Materials, resources and trained volunteers to assist women and families involved with a high-risk pregnancy.
Web: www.sidelines.org

The Society of Obstetricians and Gynaecologists of Canada
Extensive information on pregnancy, birth and postpartum.
Web: www.pregnancyinfo.ca

Spinning Babies
Videos and information to improved foetal position (breech, transverse, posterior) and birth to reduce the chance of a caesarean.
Web: www.spinningbabies.com

Star Legacy Foundation
Dedicated to reducing pregnancy loss and neonatal death and improving care for families who experience such tragedies. Involved in stillbirth research, education and awareness.
Web: www.starlegacyfoundation.org

Still Birthday
Providing support for those affected by miscarriage.
Web: www.stillbirthday.com

Still Standing Magazine
An online magazine for all who are grieving child loss and infertility.
Web: www.stillstandingmag.com

SUDC Foundation
Promotes awareness, advocates for research and supports those affected by
sudden unexpected or unexplained death in childhood.
Web: www.sudc.org

Supporting Mamas
A peer-run non-profit organisation who mission is to provide information,
resources, support and hope to women and families coping with pregnancy
and postpartum anxiety and mood disorders.
Web: www.supportingmamas.org

Through the Heart
A key resource for those experiencing pregnancy loss. A comfort kit
program and connection to resources.
Web: www.throughtheheart.org

Tiny Hands of Hope
Founded by a small group of people whose lives have been touched by the
loss of a child. Dedicated to helping families who have suffered from all
types of infant loss.
Web: www.timyhandsofhope.ca

Today's Parent
Canada's leading source for parenting content that informs, inspires and
builds a sense of community.
Web: www.todaysparent.com

WebMD
A great range of information about caring for your baby, including
development, nutrition, breastfeeding, bottle feeding and sleep.
Web: www.webmd.com/parenting/baby

What to Expect
Based on the best-selling book series, "What to Expect," this is an independent pregnancy and parenting site providing expert, authoritative and trustworthy evidence-based information on pregnancy and birth.
Web: www.whattoexpect.com

Yoga for Grief Support
Designed for individuals grieving from the death of a loved one in Edmonton, Alberta.
Web: www.yogaforgriefsupport.com

22

TERMINOLOGY INDEX

ABO Incompatibility
A type of haemolytic disease in babies where the red blood cells are broken down more quickly than usual. This can cause jaundice, anaemia and in very severe cases, death. It most often occurs with babies whose mothers have O blood type and where the baby is either A or B blood type.

Agoraphobia
An anxiety disorder that includes a fear of places and situations that might cause feelings of panic, helplessness or embarrassment.

Alagille Syndrome
This syndrome is usually diagnosed during infancy or early childhood. Alagille syndrome causes progressive destruction of the bile ducts. Over time, people with Alagille syndrome can develop liver disease.

Amniocentesis
A procedure in which amniotic fluid is removed using a hollow needle inserted into the uterus during pregnancy. The sample is used to screen for abnormalities in the developing foetus.

Amniotic Fluid
Amniotic fluid is the fluid that surrounds and protects a baby during pregnancy. This fluid contains foetal cells and various proteins.

Anaemic
The term used for a person suffering from anaemia, a condition in which you lack enough healthy red blood cells to carry adequate oxygen to your body's tissues. Having anaemia can make you feel tired and weak.

Anaphylaxis
The most severe form of allergic reaction. It is potentially life threatening and must be treated as a medical emergency requiring immediate treatment and urgent medical attention. The allergic reaction often involves more than one body system such as the skin, respiratory, gastro-intestinal and cardiovascular. It usually occurs within 20 minutes to two hours of exposure to the trigger and can rapidly become life threatening.

Angel Baby
A baby who passes away during pregnancy or shortly after birth.

Anorexia Nervosa
An eating disorder characterised by restrictive energy intake that leads to an inability to maintain what is considered a normal and healthy weight.

Anti D injection
Rhesus disease occurs during pregnancy when there is an incompatibility between the blood types of mother and baby. An antibody injection known as RH(D) Immunoglobulin or Anti D, can help prevent a woman's body from developing antibodies to their baby's blood. This helps to prevent potential harm to the baby during pregnancy and will also help to protect a woman's future pregnancies.

Anti-Müllerian Hormone (AMH) Test
Anti-Müllerian hormone is secreted by cells in developing eggs sacs (follicles) and the level of AMH in a woman's blood is a good indicator of her ovarian reserve.

Apgar Score
The Apgar score is a measure of a baby's condition after birth. It guides midwives, doctors and nurses as to whether a baby needs immediate treatment or monitoring. It is used to check a newborn baby at one minute and five minutes after their birth. It is named after Dr Virginia Apgar who developed the score.

Asthma
A medical condition that affects the airways that carry air into our lungs. People with asthma find it harder to breathe in and out because sometimes the airways in their lungs become narrower limiting the amount of air that

reaches their lungs. There is no cure for asthma, but it can be well-controlled.

Asynclitism

An asynclitic birth or asynclitism refers to the position of a foetus in the uterus such that the head of the baby is presenting first and is tilted to the shoulder, causing the foetal head to no longer be in line with the birth canal.

Australian & New Zealand Assisted Reproduction Database (ANZARD)

An initiative of the Fertility Society of Australia (FSA) to provide joint data collection for both the National Perinatal Epidemiology and Statistics Unit (NPESU) and the Reproductive Technology Accreditation Committee (RTAC) of the FSA. The purpose of ANZARD is to monitor the perinatal outcomes of assisted reproduction and to assess the effectiveness of assisted reproductive treatment.

Autism spectrum disorder (Autism)

A condition that affects a person's ability to interact with the world around them. Autism has wide-ranging levels of severity and varying characteristics. No two autistic people are alike. Autism is a neuro-developmental disability thought to have neurological or genetic causes (or both). However, the cause is not yet fully understood and there is no cure. An autistic person has difficulties in some areas of development, but other skills may develop typically.

Autoimmune Disease

A condition in which a person's immune system mistakenly attacks their body. Normally, the immune system can tell the difference between foreign cells and a person's own cells. In an autoimmune disease, the immune system mistakes part of a person's body, such as the joints or skin, as foreign.

Bicornuate Uterus

A bicornuate uterus is a type of congenital uterine malformation or müllerian duct anomaly where the uterus is heart shaped. Bicornuate uteri have two conjoined cavities whereas a typical uterus has only one cavity.

Biliary Atresia

A rare disease of the liver and bile ducts that occurs in infants. Symptoms of the disease appear or develop about two to eight weeks after birth. Cells within the liver produce liquid called bile. Bile helps to digest fat. It also carries waste products from the liver to the intestines for excretion. This network of channels and ducts is called the biliary system. When the biliary system is working the way it should, it lets the bile drain from the liver into the intestines.

When a baby has biliary atresia, bile flow from the liver to the gallbladder is blocked. This causes the bile to be trapped inside the liver, quickly causing damage and scarring of the liver cells (cirrhosis), and eventually liver failure.

Bilirubin

Bilirubin is the yellowy orange substance we all produce as we break down the haem part of the haemoglobin from our red blood cells. We change haem into unconjugated bilirubin (not water-soluble) and our livers change that unconjugated bilirubin into conjugated bilirubin (water-soluble). This conjugated bilirubin is a waste product that goes into our bile, then the intestine. It is this broken-down bilirubin in bile that gives poo its brown colour.

Braxton Hicks

These contractions are the tightenings in a woman's abdomen in preparation for giving birth. They tone the muscles of the uterus and may also help prepare the cervix for birth.

Caesarean

Also known as a c-section, this is the surgical procedure used to deliver a baby through a cut in the mother's abdomen and uterus.

Carpal Tunnel Syndrome

The carpal tunnel is a narrow passageway on the palm side of your wrist made up of bones and ligaments. The median nerve, which controls sensation and movement in the thumb and first three fingers, runs through this passageway along with tendons to the fingers and thumb. When it's pinched or compressed, the result is numbness, tingling, weakness, or pain in the hand, called carpal tunnel syndrome.

Cervical Cerclage

Also known as a cervical stitch, this is a treatments for cervical weakness when the cervix starts to shorten and open too early during a pregnancy.

Chemical Pregnancy

A term used for a very early miscarriage which occurs before the fifth week of gestation and well before the foetus can be visibly detected on an ultrasound.

Cholangiogram
A procedure where the doctor places a small tube called a catheter into the cystic duct, which drains bile from the gallbladder into the common bile duct. A dye that blocks X-rays is injected into the common bile duct, so that when the x-ray is taken, the flow of the bile can clearly be observed.

Cholangitis
Cholangitis is an inflammation of the bile duct system.

Choledochal Cysts
This is a congenital anomaly of the duct (tube) that transports bile from the liver to the gallbladder and small intestine. A choledochal cyst is a swelling of that duct that can cause bile to back up in the liver.

CIN3
Severely abnormal cells found on the surface of the cervix. Usually caused by certain types of human papillomavirus (HPV) and is found when a cervical biopsy is done. CIN 3 may become cancer and spread to nearby normal tissue if not treated.

Clomid
An ovulatory stimulating drug used to help women who have problems with ovulation.

Colic
Excessive and frequent crying in a baby who appears to be otherwise healthy and well-fed. It affects around one in five babies.

Colonoscopy
An examination of the small bowel with a camera on a flexible tube passed through the anus.

Colostrum
Colostrum is a breast fluid produced by humans, cows, and other mammals before breast milk is released. It is very nutritious and contains high levels of antibodies, which are proteins that fight infections and bacteria.

Complementary Medicine
This is the term for a group of diagnostic and therapeutic disciplines that are used together with conventional medicine. An example of a complementary therapy is being treated with acupuncture in addition to usual care to help lessen your discomfort following surgery.

Complementary medicine also includes massage therapy, hypnosis, meditation and dietary supplements.

CPAP
Continuous positive airway pressure, commonly called CPAP, is a type of respiratory support, or mechanical ventilation, used in adult and paediatric patients. In premature babies, CPAP is delivered through a set of nasal prongs or through a small mask that fits snugly over a baby's nose.

Cuddle Cot
This is a small cot specifically designed with a cooling system that effectively allows for babies who have passed away to remain with their families so that they are not required to be cooled in a mortuary environment.

D & C
This is the abbreviation for Dilation and Curettage, a procedure to remove tissue from inside the uterus.

Dermoid Cyst
These cysts can contain tissue, such as hair, skin or teeth, because they form from embryonic cells.

Diastasis Recti
A condition where a woman has the partial or complete separation of the rectus abdominis, or "six-pack" muscles, which meet at the midline of your stomach. Diastasis recti is very common during and following pregnancy. This is because the uterus stretches the muscles in the abdomen to accommodate a growing baby.

Dilation
Cervical dilation is the opening of the cervix, the entrance to the uterus, during childbirth, miscarriage, induced abortion or gynaecological surgery.

DISIDA Scan
This scan is an examination of the gallbladder and the hepatobiliary system (the ducts connecting the gallbladder to the liver and the small bowel) by injecting an intravenous radiopharmaceutical. This "tracer" is medicine combined with a small amount of radioactive material. It travels to the required area of the body and is detected and imaged by a gamma camera.

Doppler
Doppler ultrasound uses sound waves to detect the movement of blood in vessels. It is used in pregnancy to study blood circulation in the baby, uterus and placenta. It is useful to check the baby's condition in high risk pregnancies.

Doula
A doula is a non-medical labour assistant, who provides continuous physical and emotional support to the birthing woman and her partner throughout labour and birth. Doulas may also support the woman to communicate her needs and wishes to the medical team. Her key role is the creation of a birth environment which meets the woman's needs.

Down Syndrome
Down syndrome is a genetic condition where there is an extra chromosome. People with Down syndrome have 47 chromosomes in their cells instead of 46. They have an extra chromosome 21 which is why Down syndrome is sometimes known as Trisomy 21.

Echocardiography
A test that uses sound waves to produce live images of the heart. The images are called an echocardiogram. This test monitors the heart's valve functions and can help identify blood clots, fluid in the sac around the heart or problems with the aorta. It is a key tool used to determine the health of the heart muscle, including heart defects in babies.

Ectopic Pregnancy
A pregnancy in which the fertilised egg implants outside the uterus. The fertilised egg cannot survive outside the uterus and if left to grow, it can damage nearby organs causing life-threatening blood loss.

Edwards Syndrome
A genetic condition in babies that causes severe disability due to an extra copy of chromosome 18. Babies born with the condition usually do not survive for much longer than a week.

Electrocardiogram (ECG)
A medical test that detects heart abnormalities by measuring the electrical activity generated by the heart as it contracts.

Electrocardiograph
This is the machine that records a person's ECG. It displays this data as a trace on a screen or on paper.

Emergency Department (ED)

This is the department in the hospital where a person can seek urgent medical care and treatment. They are usually open 24 hours a day and have highly trained doctors and other health professionals on site to deal with emergencies.

Endocrinologist

A clinical specialist who diagnoses conditions that affect the glands. They treat hormone imbalances in the endocrine organs which include the pituitary, thyroid, adrenals, ovaries, testes and pancreas.

Endometriosis

A disorder in which the tissue that normally lines the uterus grows outside the uterus.

Endometriomas

When endometriosis involves the ovaries, fluid-filled cysts called endometriomas may form, causing pelvic pain and abnormal uterine bleeding.

Endoscopy

A procedure used in medicine to look inside the body.

ENT (Ear Nose and Throat) Specialist

A medical doctor who is a specialist in the diagnosis and treatment of disorders of the head and neck, including particularly the ears, nose, and throat. ENT doctors are also called otolaryngologists.

EPAS Clinic

EPAS is an acronym for Early Pregnancy Assessment Service. This is a dedicated outpatient service to assess, diagnose and manage women with threatened or actual early pregnancy loss, less than 20 weeks pregnant.

Epidural

An epidural is a procedure that injects a local anaesthetic into the space around the spinal nerves in your lower back. This anaesthetic usually effectively blocks the pain from labour contractions during birth.

Epigenetics

The study of biological mechanisms that will turn genes on and off. It involves genetic control by factors other than an individual's DNA sequence.

Epilepsy

A disease of the brain where there is a tendency to have recurrent seizures. It is a neurological disorder, not a form of mental illness, and seizures are caused by a temporary disruption of the electrical activity in the brain.

Episiotomy

An episiotomy is a surgical cut at the opening of the vagina during childbirth to aid a difficult delivery and to prevent the rupture of tissue.

Examination Under Anaesthetic (EUA)

This is an internal examination under general anaesthetic. The test is used to visually examine the area of concern. The doctor may take tissue samples during the test if necessary.

Exploding Head Syndrome

These are loud, explosion-like noises that an affected person hears when drifting off to sleep or when waking up. They are a type of hallucination that though imagined, feel very real. The noises can jolt a person awake and keep them from falling asleep. They can happen only once or be a recurring experience and typically happen between sleep stages.

Facet Joint

Facet joints are located between the individual vertebrae of the spine and help to support the body's weight and control movement. Facet joint injury occurs when the connective tissue or cartilage surrounding the joint becomes damaged or tears when an excessive force is placed on it.

Fibromyalgia

A disorder characterised by widespread musculoskeletal pain accompanied by fatigue, sleep, memory and mood issues. Researchers believe that fibromyalgia amplifies painful sensations by affecting the way your brain processes pain signals. Symptoms sometime start after a physical trauma, surgery, infection or severe psychological stress. In other cases, symptoms gradually accumulate over time with no single triggering event.

Fluoroscopy

An imaging technique that uses x-rays to obtain real-time images of the body.

Foley's Bulb

Also referred to as Foley's catheter, this is an induction method where a doctor insets a catheter into the mother's cervix. One side of the catheter is deflated. Once inside the womb, the doctor inflates the balloon with a saline solution to put pressure on the cervix and encourage dilation in preparation for birth.

Forceps
An instrument shaped like a large pair of spoons or salad tongs. It is applied to a baby's head to help guide the baby out of the birth canal.

Gas
A pain relief option during labour. The gas is a mixture of nitrous oxide mixed with oxygen and is also called Entonox or just gas. It is safe for mother and baby.

Gastroenterologist
A medical practitioner qualified to diagnose and treat disorders of the stomach and intestines.

General Practitioner
Australia, NZ, Europe and the UK refer to the family doctor as a General Practitioner. In the USA and Canada, the equivalent term is Family Physician (FP) or Family Medicine (FM).

Gestational Diabetes
A condition characterised by elevated levels of glucose (sugar) in their blood during pregnancy. It typically resolves after birth.

Glucose Tolerance Test (GTT)
A test to measure how well your body's cells are able to absorb glucose (sugar) after you consume a specific amount of sugar.

Grommets
Grommets are tiny tubes which are inserted into the eardrum. They allow air to pass through the eardrum in order to keep the air pressure on either side equal. The grommet usually stays in place for six to 12 months and then falls out.

Harmony Test
The Harmony prenatal test is a non-invasive screening test that looks at fragments of your baby's DNA to provide accurate information about the likelihood of the most common chromosomal conditions.

Heartfelt Photography
A volunteer organisation of professional photographers from all over Australia and New Zealand, dedicated to giving the gift of photographic

memories to families that have experienced stillbirths, premature births or have children with serious and terminal illnesses.

Human Chorionic Gonadotropin (hCG) Levels

Human chorionic gonadotropin (hCG) is a hormone normally produced by the placenta. When a woman is pregnant, it can be detected in the urine. Blood tests measuring hCG levels can also be used to check the progress of a pregnancy.

HELLP syndrome

An acronym for Haemolysis, Elevated Liver enzymes Low Platelet count, HELLP Syndrome is rare but serious complication in pregnancy that is usually associated with pre-eclampsia. It is a disorder of the liver and blood that is potentially life-threatening for mother and baby if left untreated.

Haemorrhagic Ovarian Cyst

When an internal haemorrhage occurs inside functional ovarian cysts.

Hepatobiliary System

The body system that includes the liver, gallbladder, bile ducts, or bile.

Hip Dysplasia

Observed in babies and sometimes in children around the time they are learning to walk, hip dysplasia is sometimes called 'clicky hips' because when you move the hips of babies with this condition, you can often feel a little click. In a normal baby, the ball at the top of their thighbone (the femoral head) is held in a cup-shaped socket in the pelvis. The ball is held in in the socket by ligaments and muscles. When a baby has hip dysplasia, the femoral head has moved away from the normal position and requires them to wear a brace to correct.

Honestly Store

An online store created by Adele where customers can purchase scientifically researched natural and aromatherapy products for mothers and babies. www.honestlystore.com.au

HPV 16 and 18

HPV is short for human papillomavirus, a common virus that infects nearly everyone at some point. HPV 16 and 18 have been shown to significantly increase the risk of cervical cancer as well as genital cancers.

Hydrocephalus

The abnormal enlargement of the brain cavities (ventricles) caused by a build-up of cerebrospinal fluid (CSF). Usually, the body maintains a constant circulation and absorption of CSF. Untreated, hydrocephalus can result in brain damage or death. There is no cure, but hydrocephalus can be managed with surgery.

Hyperemesis
Nausea and vomiting are common in pregnancy, especially in the first trimester. Some pregnant women experience excessive nausea and vomiting. This condition is known as 'hyperemesis gravidarum' and often needs hospital treatment.

Hysterectomy
The surgical removal of the uterus. It may also involve removal of the cervix, fallopian tubes and other surrounding structures.

Incision Biopsy
A procedure in which a sample of suspicious tissue is cut from the body and removed for diagnostic purposes.

Intensive Care Unit (ICU)
A special department in a hospital for acutely unwell patients who require critical medical care.

Intrauterine Insemination (IUI)
A fertility treatment that involves placing sperm inside a woman's uterus to facilitate fertilisation. The goal of IUI is to increase the number of sperm that reach the fallopian tubes and subsequently increase the chance of fertilisation.

In Utero
This is the term used to describe a woman's uterus before the birth of her baby.

Intravenous Therapy (IV)
This is a therapy that delivers fluids directly into a vein. It can be used to administer injections using a syringe as well as infusions.

In Vitro Fertilisation (IVF)
A medical procedure whereby an egg is fertilised by sperm outside of the body. It involves monitoring and stimulating a woman's ovulatory process, harvesting ova and fertilising them with sperm in a laboratory to create an embryo.

Irritable Bowel Syndrome (IBS)
An intestinal disorder causing pain in the stomach, wind, diarrhoea and constipation.

Jaundice
A condition in newborn infants that affects both full-term and premature babies, usually appearing during the first week of the baby's life. It normally happens when there is a build-up of a naturally occurring substance in the blood called bilirubin, an orange/red pigment in the blood. Bilirubin is produced by the normal breakdown of red blood cells. As bilirubin begins to build up, it deposits on the fatty tissue under the skin causing the baby's skin and whites of the eyes to appear yellow.

Kasai Procedure
This procedure involves removing the blocked bile ducts and gallbladder and replacing them with a small segment of the child's own small intestine. This segment of intestine is sewn to the liver and provides a new path that can allow bile to drain from the liver.

Ketamine
A medication mainly used for starting and maintaining anaesthesia. It induces a trance-like state while providing pain relief, sedation, and memory loss. Other uses include sedation in intensive care and treatment of pain and depression.

Laparoscopy
A surgical procedure that allows a surgeon to access the inside of the abdomen and pelvis without having to make large incisions in the skin. It is also known as keyhole surgery.

Laparotomy
A surgical procedure involving a large incision through the abdominal wall to gain access into the abdominal cavity.

Large for Gestational Age (LGA)
A term used to describe newborn babies who weigh significantly more than the average weight for their number of weeks of pregnancy. Babies may be called LGA if they weigh more than 9 in 10 babies (90th percentile) or more than 97 of 100 babies (97th percentile) of the same gestational age.

Large Loop Excision of the Transformation Zone (LLETZ)
Also called loop electrosurgical excision procedure (LEEP), this is the most common way of removing cervical tissue for examination and treatment

of precancerous cells of the cervix. The abnormal tissue is removed using a thin wire loop that is heated electrically.

Lumber Puncture
Also known as a spinal tap, this is a medical procedure in which a needle is inserted into the spinal canal to collect and remove a sample of cerebrospinal fluid for diagnostic testing.

Lymphoedema
Swelling in an arm or leg caused by a lymphatic system blockage.

Lymphoma
This refers to types of cancer that begin in the lymphatic system. When you have lymphoma, large numbers of abnormal lymphocytes are made and some of these replace your normal lymphocytes. This can affect you immune system and lymph nodes can become swollen forming lumps (tumours).

Maya Abdominal/Womb Massage
A non-invasive, external massage that repositions internal organs that have shifted and restricted the flow of blood, lymph, nerve impulses and chi. It can enhance pregnancy and aids in labour and delivery.

Meconium
The term for a newborn's first poo. This sticky, thick, dark green poo is made up of cells, protein, fats, and intestinal secretions, like bile.

Meconium Aspiration Syndrome (MAS)
A condition that occurs when a newborn infant breathes in a mixture of meconium and amniotic fluid. The inhaled meconium can partially or completely block the baby's airways, making it difficult for the infant to breath, causing irritation or a lung infection. It can also prevent the normal function of an important lung chemical called surfactant, which helps the lungs expand properly.

Medically Managed Miscarriage
Sometimes the symptoms of miscarriage, including bleeding and/or pain, are not immediately obvious. Medical management uses medication to speed up the process of miscarriage.

Medical Emergency Team (MET)
The MET call is part of a Rapid Response System used in hospitals. It is designed for staff members to alert and call other staff for help when a patient's vital signs have fallen outside set criteria.

Membrane Sweep
A method to induce labour where the doctor sweeps a gloved finger between the thin membranes of the amniotic sac and the mother's uterus. The motion helps separate the sac and stimulates prostaglandins, compounds that act like hormones and bring on labour.

Meningitis
Inflammation of brain and spinal cord membranes, typically caused by an infection.

Metformin
Marketed under the trade name Glucophage among others. This is the first-line medication for the treatment of Type 2 diabetes, particularly in people who are overweight. It is also used in the treatment of polycystic ovary syndrome.

Methylenetetrahydrofolate Reductase (MTHFR)
A genetic mutation that may lead to high levels of homocysteine (an amino acid produced when proteins are broken down) and low levels of folate and other vitamins. Research is currently evolving and may be linked to recurrent miscarriages.

Midwifery Group Practice (MGP)
MGP offers pregnant women with low risk factors, the continuity of care from one midwife with the support of a team if he/she is not available. It also offers the option of home birth for some women.

Mobile Intensive Care Ambulance (MICA) Paramedic
MICA paramedics have a higher clinical skill set than general paramedics and can perform more advanced medical procedures.

Midazolam
A drug used before surgery or a procedure to cause drowsiness, decrease anxiety and to decrease your memory of the surgery or procedure. Midazolam works by calming the brain and nerves. It belongs to a class of drugs known as benzodiazepines.

MoMo Twins
Monoamniotic twins are identical and share the same amniotic sac within their mother's uterus. Monoamniotic twins are always identical, always monochorionic and are usually termed Monoamniotic-Monochorionic ("MoMo" or "Mono Mono") twins. They share the placenta but have two separate umbilical cords.

Mucus Plug

The mucus plug is a protective collection of mucus in the cervical canal. During pregnancy, the cervix secretes a thick, jelly-like fluid to keep the area moist and protected. This fluid eventually accumulates and seals the cervical canal, creating a thick plug of mucus. The mucus plug acts as a barrier and can keep unwanted bacteria and other sources of infection from travelling into the uterus. Losing a mucus plug during pregnancy can be a precursor to childbirth. As the cervix begins to open wider in preparation for delivery, the mucus plug is discharged into the vagina.

Nasogastric Tube (NGT)

A thin, soft tube that is passed through a child's nostril, down the back of their throat, through the oesophagus and into their stomach.

Newborn & Paediatric Emergency Transport Service (NETS)

A state-wide service of NSW Health that is hosted by the Sydney Children's Hospitals Network. It is the only service of its kind in Australia and provides expert clinical advice and co-ordination, emergency treatment and inter-hospital transport for very sick babies and children up to the age of 16 years. The service operates 24/7.

Natural Killer Cells (NK Cells)

These are a type of lymphocyte (a white blood cell) and a component of the innate immune system. NK cells play a major role in the host-rejection of both tumours and virally infected cells.

Neonatal Intensive Care Unit (NICU)

A hospital intensive care unit that specialises in looking after premature and sick newborn babies.

Non-Invasive Prenatal Test (NIPT)

A highly sensitive test that screens for Down Syndrome and certain other abnormalities in a baby.

Nuchal Translucency Scan

A scan that is part of the ultrasound scan that most pregnant women have at around 12 weeks of pregnancy. The sonographer performing the ultrasound will measure the size of the nuchal fold at the back of a baby's neck. The results may tell you if the baby has a high or low risk of a chromosomal abnormality.

Obstructive Sleep Apnoea

This is the intermittent airflow blockage during sleep. Symptoms include snoring and daytime sleepiness.

Oxytocin
A hormone produced by the hypothalamus and secreted by the pituitary gland. It is responsible for signalling contractions of the womb during labour. It is administered to start labour or speed up labour.

Panadol
Panadol is the brand name for paracetamol, a medication used to treat pain and fever. It is typically used for mild to moderate pain relief.

Patent Ductus Arteriosus (PDA)
This condition is a heart defect found in the days or weeks after birth. The ductus arteriosus is a normal part of foetal blood circulation before a baby is born. It is an extra blood vessel that connects two arteries: the pulmonary artery and the aorta. The pulmonary artery carries blood from the heart to the lungs. The aorta carries blood from the heart to the body. Before birth, the ductus arteriosus lets blood bypass the lungs. This is because the baby gets oxygen from the mother. All babies are born with this opening between the aorta and the pulmonary artery, but it normally closes on its own shortly after birth, once the baby breathes on its own. If it stays open it is PDA. Extra blood flows to the lungs and if the PDA is large, too much blood goes to the lungs. The blood vessels and the lungs have to work much harder to handle the extra blood. This can lead to fluid build-up in the lungs making it harder for the baby to breathe and feed.

Patent Foramen Ovale (PFO)
A hole in the heart in the wall between the left and right atria. When a baby is born and takes its first breath, the foramen ovale closes and within a few months it has sealed completely in around 75% of people. For the millions of adults with PFO, it is generally not a problem except in cases where the blood contains a blood clot.

Patient-Controlled Analgesia (PCA)
This term describes any method of allowing a person in pain to administer their own pain relief through an infusion programmed by medical staff.

Perinatal
Pertaining to the period immediately before or after birth.

PET Scan
An image made using Positron Emission Tomography (PET) techniques that use radioactive substances to visualise and measure metabolic processes in the body.

Phlebotomist
A phlebotomist draws blood from patients for research, testing, transfusions or donation.

Phototherapy
This is a treatment that uses light to eliminate bilirubin in the blood. A baby's skin and blood absorb these light waves that change bilirubin into products which can processed and passed through the infant's system.

Placenta Accreta
A serious pregnancy condition that occurs when the placenta grows too deeply into the uterine wall. Typically, the placenta detaches from the uterine wall after childbirth. With placenta accreta, part or all of the placenta remains attached. This can cause severe blood loss after delivery. It's also possible for the placenta to invade the muscles of the uterus (placenta increta) or grow through the uterine wall (placenta percreta). Placenta accreta is considered a high-risk pregnancy complication.

Placenta Chronic Villitis
This is a placental injury. It is an inflammatory condition that can be recurrent and can also be associated with intrauterine growth restriction.

Placenta Praevia
When the placenta covers the opening in the mother's cervix. The condition can cause severe bleeding and can interfere with the vaginal delivery of a baby.

Polycystic Ovary Syndrome (PCOS)
A set of symptoms related to a hormonal imbalance that can affect women and girls of reproductive age.

Polymyalgia
An inflammatory disorder causing muscle pain and stiffness around the shoulders and hips.

Postnatal Anxiety
Symptoms can include feelings of anxiety and stress that won't go away, panic, agoraphobia, and obsessive-compulsive disorder, PTSD and social phobia.

Postnatal Depression (PND)
A type of depression that comes on within 12 months of having a baby, usually during the first few weeks or months. It can start slowly or suddenly, and can range from very mild and transient, to severe and

lingering. For some women it passes quickly, but others will need professional help.

Postpartum Psychosis
Postpartum psychosis is a serious mental illness that can develop in mothers soon after childbirth, causing major changes in mood and behaviour. The condition can come on very suddenly, sometimes within hours of giving birth. The word 'psychosis' refers to a loss of sense of reality. Symptoms may include seeing or hearing things that are not there (hallucinations), feeling everyone is against you (paranoia) and powerful delusions (beliefs that clearly conflict with reality). Women with postpartum psychosis need specialised psychiatric treatment to get better.

Post-Traumatic Stress Disorder (PTSD)
A set of reactions that can occur after someone has experienced trauma. Symptoms include reliving events, avoiding reminders, negative thoughts and feelings, depression and anxiety.

Pre-eclampsia
A serious condition of pregnancy that can be life-threatening to both mother and unborn child, characterised by high blood pressure, protein in the urine and severe swelling.

Pre-term Birth
Also called premature birth, this refers to birth that takes place more than three weeks before the baby's estimated due date.

Premature Labour
When a pregnant woman goes into labour with contractions starting more than three weeks before the baby's estimated due date.

Posterior
The OP position (occiput posterior foetal position) is when the back of baby's head is against the mother's back.

Pulmonary Stenosis
A condition where the pulmonary valve (the valve between the right ventricle and the pulmonary artery) is too small, narrow or stiff.

Rainbow Baby
A baby born after a miscarriage, stillbirth or neonatal death. The name represents hope.

Reflux

Infant reflux occurs when food backs up from a baby's stomach causing the infant to spit up.

Salpingectomy

The surgical removal of one or both fallopian tubes.

Sever's Disease

Also known as calcaneal apophysitis, this is one of the most common causes of heel pain in growing children and adolescents. It is an inflammation of the growth plate in the calcaneus (heel). Sever's disease is caused by repetitive stress to the heel, and most often occurs during growth spurts, when bones, muscles, tendons, and other structures are changing rapidly.

Silent Reflux

A condition in which stomach acid causes throat discomfort. Refluxed material flows back into the oesophagus but isn't forced out of the mouth.

Sleep Apnoea

A sleep disorder where a person has pauses in breathing or periods of shallow breathing during sleep. Each pause can last for a few seconds to a few minutes and they happen many times a night. In the most common form, this follows loud snoring.

Sonogram

Also known as an ultrasound, A pregnancy ultrasound is a test that uses high-frequency sound waves to image the developing baby. It is used to monitor normal foetal development and screen for any potential problems.

Sperm Washing

Sperm washing is a procedure to prepare sperm for intrauterine insemination (IUI) or in vitro fertilisation (IVF). It aims to remove chemicals from the semen which may cause adverse reactions in the female's uterus. During the sperm washing process, individual sperms are separated from the seminal fluid. It not only extracts certain disease-carrying material in the semen but also enhances the fertilising capacity of the sperm.

Split Bilirubin Blood Test

This test checks a baby's blood for the ratio of conjugated (not water-soluble) and unconjugated (water soluble) bilirubin. The conjugated bilirubin is a waste product that goes into the baby's bile, then into the intestine. It is this broken-down bilirubin in bile that gives a baby's poo a brown colour. The test helps to determine whether or not a baby's jaundice is caused by an underlying condition such as biliary atresia or liver disease.

Subchorionic Haematoma
A condition where there is an accumulation of blood between the uterine lining and the chorion (the outer foetal membrane, next to the uterus) or under the placenta itself. It can cause light to heavy spotting or bleeding, but it may not.

Sunshine Baby
A baby born before a miscarriage, still birth, infant death or other early loss of a child. The name represents the calm before.

Syntocinon
A drug that can be used to induce labour or during and immediately after delivery to help the birth and to prevent or treat excessive bleeding. Syntocinon is a man-made chemical that is identical to a natural hormone called oxytocin. It works by stimulating the muscles of the uterus to produce rhythmic contractions.

Tongue-tie
Also called Ankyloglossia, tongue-tie is a condition in which the thin piece of skin under the baby's tongue (lingual frenulum) is abnormally short and may restrict the movement of the tongue.

Trachelectomy
The surgical removal of the cervix, the lower portion of the uterus that protrudes into the vagina. Trachelectomys are performed on younger women with early cancer of the cervix.

Transcutaneous Bilirubinometer
A device which measures the yellowness of the subcutaneous tissue by directing white light into the skin of a newborn and measuring the intensity of specific wavelengths that are returned. From this information the concentration of bilirubin can be determined.

Trisomy 15
Chromosome 15, Distal Trisomy 15q is an extremely rare chromosomal disorder in which the end (distal) portion of the long arm (q) of the 15th chromosome (15q) appears three times (trisomy) rather than twice in cells of the body. The disorder is characterised by growth delays before and/or after birth; mental retardation; and/or distinctive malformations of the head and facial (craniofacial) area.

Trisomy 18
Children with Trisomy 18 have three copies of part or all of chromosome 18, instead of the usual two copies. It is also called Edwards Syndrome, a genetic condition in babies that causes severe disabilities. Babies with this condition do not usually survive for much longer than a week.

Turner's Syndrome
A random genetic disorder that affects females. The main characteristics include short stature and infertility. A female usually has two X chromosomes, but in females with Turner's Syndrome, one of these chromosomes are missing or abnormal. It is estimated that only one percent of foetuses with this abnormality survive to term and as many as 10 percent of miscarriages have this chromosomal abnormality.

Type 2 Diabetes
Type 2 diabetes is a progressive condition in which the body becomes resistant to the normal effects of insulin and/or gradually loses the capacity to produce enough insulin in the pancreas.

Ultrasound
Also known as a sonogram, a pregnancy ultrasound is a test that uses high-frequency sound waves to image the developing baby. It is used to monitor normal foetal development and screen for any potential problem.

Uterine Atony
Atony of the uterus, also called uterine atony, is a serious condition that can occur after childbirth. It occurs when the uterus fails to contract after the delivery of a baby, and it can lead to a potentially life-threatening condition known as postpartum haemorrhage.

Vega Machine
A type of electroacupuncture device used to diagnose allergies and illnesses.

Vaginal Birth after Caesarean (VBAC)
A vaginal birth by a woman who has undergone a caesarean section in a previous pregnancy.

Ventouse Vacuum Assisted Delivery
This is a delivery method that uses a vacuum device to help guide a baby out of the birth canal. The vacuum device, known as a vacuum extractor, uses a soft cup that attaches to your baby's head with suction.

ENJOY THIS BOOK?

Would you like to help the millions of women and families around the world affected by pregnancy, infant loss, premature and sick newborns?

By getting the word out about this book, more women will feel less isolated. Reading these relatable and inspiring stories will show them that others have survived and revived so they can too.

A great way you can assist is through honest reviews. This simple act will bring this book to the attention of those seeking this knowledge.

I would be grateful if you could spend a few minutes leaving a review on the page where you purchased this book, such as Amazon, Apple Books or your favourite online book store. It can be as short as you like and your efforts are much appreciated.

ABOUT THE AUTHOR

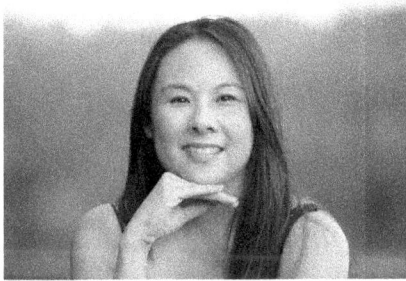

Jo Spicer is an author, speaker and advocate who uses her own lived experience to help others overcome the devastating effects of trauma. A survivor of two cancers, the traumatic pregnancy and births of her two children, debilitating migraines, financial crisis, two divorces, emotional abuse and PTSD, Jo had to find ways to deal with both physical and emotional wounds.

Through her personal journey and her research with other survivors, Jo has discovered the secrets to processing and overcoming trauma. She has developed strategies that resonate strongly with others. She has learnt to thrive and now lives with the purpose of helping those who are struggling, offering practical guidance and real hope to light their way forward.

Find out more about Jo and her inspirational books, quotes, art, handmade original gifts and homewares at www.brightbutterfly.com.au

facebook.com/brightbfly

twitter.com/brightbfly

instagram.com/brightbfly

www.ingramcontent.com/pod-product-compliance
Lightning Source LLC
Chambersburg PA
CBHW060027030426
42334CB00019B/2220